© Copyright 2022 Intuitive Way Publishing - All rights reserved.

The content contained within this book may not be reproduced, duplicated or transmitted without direct written permission from the author or the publisher. Under no circumstances will any blame or legal responsibility be held against the publisher, or author, for any damages, reparation, or monetary loss due to the information contained within this book, either directly or indirectly.

Legal Notice:

This book is copyright protected. It is only for personal use. You cannot amend, distribute, sell, use, quote or paraphrase any part, or the content within this book, without the consent of the author or publisher.

Disclaimer Notice:

Please note the information contained within this document is for educational and entertainment purposes only. All effort has been executed to present accurate, up to date, reliable, complete information. No warranties of any kind are declared or implied. Readers acknowledge that the author is not engaged in the rendering of legal, financial, medical or professional advice. The content within this book has been derived from various sources. Please consult a licensed professional before attempting any techniques outlined in this book.

By reading this document, the reader agrees that under no circumstances is the author responsible for any losses, direct or indirect, that are incurred as a result of the use of the information contained within this document, including, but not limited to, errors, omissions, or inaccuracies.

Editor: Nigel Lavers

Intuitive Way Publishing is a division of Hedhaus Inc

158F Brairwynd Court, Edmonton, AB, Canada, T5T 0H4

ISBN: 9798834295891

Cover art: UnSplash.com

www.intuitive-way.com

INTUITIVE WAY

Contents

Book 1 – Trauma Healing Workbook

Trauma Healing Workbook

A Bottom-up Approach to Healing From C-PTSD

Dan Hartman

INTRODUCTION

Happiness can be found in the darkest of times if only one remembers to turn on the light.

- J. K. Rowling

As a behavioral medicine practitioner, I am blessed to come in contact with people from all walks of life. Everyone is governed by their traumas—those who handle them to rise above, triumph in life; those who don't, unfortunately, sing the same sad song every day. How people deal with this trauma is what decides how their life shapes up. With the practices taught in this book, we will learn to adopt the attitude of healing, and to incorporate habits of love into our lives. With these practices we will learn to cultivate our emotional intelligence. This will strengthen our resolve to right ourselves from the past wrongs and past traumas—to start singing a new tune, one of harmony and abundant joy.

When these traumatic experiences unravel in our lives, it's easy to quickly lose hope. In that moment, it's even natural to feel like things will never be okay. The reality remains, however, that without working through these traumas consciously, they likely continue to overpower our psyche. The only way to be free of this power struggle is to bring these traumatic experiences out in the open through a gradual process of dissolution. What ensues is a conscious awakening—an authentic breakthrough.

Specializing in behavioral medicine, I am concerned with the prevention, diagnosis, treatment, and rehabilitation of anyone who is suffering from past and present trauma as well as a threat of future traumas. One thing I observed, though, is that the presence of a therapist is hardly the most important aspect of this healing. I've been a witness to individuals breaking the shackles of their past trauma all on their own while I act as an observer, a guide, a signpost. This healing power they exhibit is a mixture of an individual's conscious awareness and their desire to be free from the bondages of pain and suffering.

The trauma we experience may come from one or more of the most common sources:

1. Physical or emotional neglect where our physical and emotional needs were never acknowledged or fulfilled.

2. Physical or emotional abuse in the form of corporal punishment, gaslighting, bullying, derision, and so on.

3. Sexual abuse involving unwanted exposure to sexually explicit images and experiences, unconsented touching, molestation, and rape.

4. Catastrophes like natural disasters, exposure to war, accidents, and the like, leading to the loss of a loved one or an important aspect of our life.

When any of these traumas are repressed, they're likely to develop into a condition known as post-traumatic stress disorder (PTSD). Having worked with people experiencing this, I've come to realize that regardless of what stage of life we are in, whether we are children (in memory), adolescent, an adult, or someone in their old age, trauma has a pattern of manifestation that is similar across racial and ethnic backgrounds. When traumas are inflicted upon children, they start off as adverse childhood experiences (ACEs) which, like unaddressed PTSD, can lead to a complex of traumas and ensuing behaviors to accommodate these additional stresses.

As a mental health counselor, I have observed the hampering influence of trauma on effectiveness in preventing and healing from disease. If left unattended, traumas may very well impede our ability to live a full and content life. Even though it may seem that the trauma fades with time, they can come back in a full-blown manner when brought face-to-face with certain triggers in our environment. Through lifestyle change, training, and social support, we can develop and implement successful behavior changes to recover from complex post-traumatic stress disorder (C-PTSD) and achieve resolution.

Written in a didactic sense, this workbook aims to enable us, the readers, to move from uncertainty in our mind to clarity in our hearts. We will discover that through a series of exercises, we can become fully prepared for a future of health and healing. By following through with the exercises in this workbook, we will find splendor and bravery within ourselves. Let us now affirm this together:

"I am born for this. I am prepared to live a life of splendor and bravery."

This workbook is divided into four parts, each requiring about 5 days to complete. Of course, anyone could finish the whole book in one afternoon, but before we try that, I recommend giving ourselves the time to properly digest everything and witness the changes in our lives. In the end, it might take up to 60 days for any new indications of change to emerge in our daily routine, but the results we achieve in this workbook will be marked as a keystone in a bridge to becoming resolved in our healing journey.

This is what we'll need to accommodate the exercises—a pad of paper, a blue or black pen, and some color crayons with at least seven different colors.

PART I

CHAPTER 1: DISARM AND REAFFIRM

The darkest nights produce the brightest stars.

- John Green

My favorite memory of my twin sons is when they were both in their highchairs and we would try to feed them solid foods—what a mess! But with enough practice, we learned to clean up after them and get them fed. Much like a baby's reflex to hold onto a rattle with surprising strength, we too have natural instincts that are simultaneously innocent and powerful. It's important to explore these as best as we can. And just as we learned to handle our kids, anyone can learn to manage their instincts for a healthy and happy life.

While these instincts keep us protected, they also keep us holding on to the trauma because it is still a piece of our life that we are familiar with. Until, and unless, we explore the instinct holding on to our PTSD, we can make no real headway. So, let's begin this process, unearth the instinct that's holding us back, and learn to release it without fear of the colorful mess it'll make when it drops to the floor.

THE COLOR OF EMOTIONS

This is what we are going to do. We're going to put words to our emotions—something we have rarely done, especially when it comes to our traumas. This can be overwhelming at times. So, it is a good recommendation that we pace ourselves. If at any point we feel overcome with emotion, stop the activity and try again when the feeling is truly comfortable.

This is why I previously said it's important to not just breeze through this workbook but take the time to digest it. When we still feel unsettled, it's easy to simply reach out for help from loved ones and even a professional.

Sit in a calm place, without any interruptions, with the writing pad, pen, and crayons. Now, without going into the specifics of our trauma, we focus on the feeling(s) that it provokes. Using words like "anger," "pain," "grief," "sadness," "annoyance," and so forth, we write out anywhere on the blank page all the emotions that come to mind when we think of the trauma. We can use the names of the people who were with us, the place where it occurred, the time of day, and the sounds we heard or words we used while it happened.

Use at least 10 words, preferably more. Next, go back and place a number between 1 and 5 right next to the word—5 being the worst and 1 being not so bad. Finally, with our colored crayons we just color over the words with any color we like so that the word appears vividly on the page.

Now, as we can see, the power of these emotions has been triggered, and we're aware of the trigger results—in the past they were unbearable, but today they are mere numbers and colors. Our instincts to digest, breathe, move, laugh, play, and generally enjoy life are tied up in these words, and we are going to set ourselves free from them, one by one, day by day.

CHAPTER 2: YOUR INSTINCTS, YOUR LIFE

The workings of the amygdala and its interplay with the neocortex are at the heart of emotional intelligence.

- Daniel Goleman

Much of how we initially react to our personal traumatic experiences comes from the biological standpoint. The fight-or-flight response is a product of our sympathetic nervous system giving bursts of energy to help us survive, driven by the amygdala in our brain. This gland is part of what manages fear and stress, but it is also pivotal in its role with memory.

In ancient times, this response served the purpose of keeping us safe from physical dangers. Today we live in a different world—our dangers are not so much physical anymore, but very much psychological in nature. Though even today, this response, sometimes called the adrenaline rush, is necessary for us to cope with sudden crises, the continued stimulation of this pathway can be quite obtrusive for our general well-being. Unfortunately, C-PTSD continues to trigger the amygdala, delivering a short circuit of elevated stress hormones like cortisol, producing a consequent loss of our ability to control our emotions. This instinct greatly heightens the risk of heart disease and stroke and needs to be tamed before it overwhelms our daily lives.

Disarming the fight-or-flight response from C-PTSD symptoms lets our baby-like instincts grow and experience life again, in an innocent way. This is a practice of mindfulness. Now, instead of combating these words and the impressions that come with them, we reaffirm our instincts which we have been using to protect ourselves and prevent them from short-circuiting again. This is achieved by reaffirming this dominion over our instincts through relaxation, and by learning to enjoy the fruits of relaxation with laughter—the best medicine.

I reaffirm with you now—no matter the past, you are still the one in charge. And fear not, to laugh in the face of trauma is not just the labor of heroes and heroines, but of everyday people. The testimony of those millions who have healed from trauma is their gratitude for life.

LAUGH IT OFF

Sit in a relaxed position, again without any interruptions. Make sure your body is relaxed. If you are feeling stiff in any part of your body, just assume a posture that feels the most natural to you. Use comfortable soothing music, nothing too jarring and distracting. Breathing normally, start curling the edges of your mouth, up and down, and then let a smile form on your face. Pay attention to the change the smile brings in your mood. Enjoy the smile and after a while, it's highly likely that it will not feel forced.

Now, onto the next step—as you start feeling comfortable smiling for no reason, laugh for no reason, too. It's fine if you need to force it in the beginning but eventually, and this might take a while, the real laughter will follow. Be aware of the joyous sensation in your stomach, chest, face, and rest of your body as well. This is what joy feels like—let your entire being soak in it for as long as you wish.

PART II

CHAPTER 3: REASSOCIATE AND REVITALIZE

You can't turn a screw with a hammer.

- Unknown

After experiencing the triumph of our ringing beautiful laughter, we may be tempted to feel like we are healed, like our trauma can never overpower us again. Well, we're not there yet. But we've just begun the journey of a lifetime, and we are only going to gain strength at every step from here on out. It's true that we haven't overcome all of it, but we're well on our way. But while laughter brings joy to us, it doesn't necessarily address the negative feelings buried within. And hence, to turn the screw of our repressed negative feelings, we just need something greater than the hammer of laughter.

Have you ever wondered why, after all that elapsed time, a trigger can bring back your trauma as if it happened yesterday? It's because of the associations that we formed. A person can bring back the memory of abuse, a car can bring back the memory of that horrible accident we were in, the triggers could be anything. It's unnerving knowing our trauma can return anytime a trigger is encountered in our environment.

But the good news about these associations is that if they were formed once, they can be formed again. We can reassociate our words, thoughts, and deeds to the world around us in a new way. And we can also revitalize ourselves with a daily recharge to improve the certainty of our goals. What's the goal? Well, it's precisely the happiness and innocence we so desire.

THE MUSICAL SCALE

Sit comfortably with eyes closed to keep away from distractions. Now, we imagine on the screen of our mind the notes on a scale—do, rey, mi, fa, so, la, ti, do. The scale is vertical and starts with 'do' at the bottom but also finishes with 'do' at the top!

Now visualize the negative emotions we spoke of in Chapter 1 in the color we used to color them. Each time we visualize the color of the negative emotion rising up the scale, let it slowly turn to white and fade away to clear. This can be done for every word and color we wrote down on the page.

It is possible to do this before bedtime at the end of the day, in the safety and comfort of our bed, or in the morning just after waking up. If the color refuses to fade away to clear after white, simply repeat the scale by going another octave up using the inner ear. We should take our time until every word on the page has been cleared. Again, the speed at which we clear all the words is of much less significance than the fact that we are doing it. So, let's take the time and let these words be released from our system at our own pace.

CHAPTER 4: CHANGE YOUR FUEL (I)

As we move forward on our journey, we may realize that triggers have a way of sneaking up on us. We may not have realized or identified some of them before, but they still surprise us every now and then with the intensity they come at us with. There may also be some trigger words from our list we haven't released from our system. In both these cases, we need a ***backup*** while we continue to scan our environments for new triggers and try the musical scale visualization technique to clear out the existing ones. We might be surprised to know that ***backup*** exists right within us.

When our C-PTSD overcomes our sympathetic nervous system (SNS) we experience inconsistencies in our breath. Acclimatizing to the power of breathing has the power to free us from the shock of any triggers which haven't yet dissolved through the clearing process.

In the coming exercise, we'll explore what is called a cosmic breath. Much like the cosmos expands and contracts over billions and billions of years, our body too is undergoing expansion and contraction as we breathe. This life breath is the fuel of our soul. Without this cosmic breath, our blood wouldn't be able to drive any activity to our stomach and our food wouldn't digest, starving our brain and muscles from nourishment.

The air we breathe is our fuel, and the mechanism to bring this into our bodies is through the windpipe and the lungs. Cosmic breathing awakens the universe within us, so that the rewiring of our hippocampus and prefrontal cortex occurs everywhere we use this conscious form of breath. We regain rationality and control.

THE POWER OF A COSMIC BREATH

For the cosmic breathing exercise, just sit in a place without any disruptions. We should take in a deep breath through the nose and feel our belly and our chest expanding and contracting. Be aware of the connection that we have right in that moment to our physical as well as spiritual core. We should focus on the breath as much as possible, letting it be fluid, in and out. When our attention moves to anxious thoughts, we simply bring it back to our breath. When we repeat this as many times as we need, we eventually learn to calm our anxieties, day over day, week over week, month over month.

CHAPTER 5: CHANGE YOUR FUEL (II)

There is a battle of two wolves inside us all. One is evil—it is anger, jealousy, greed, resentment, inferiority, lies, and ego. The other is good—it is joy, peace, love, hope, humility, kindness, empathy, and truth. The wolf that wins is the one you feed.

- Cherokee Proverb

It's crucial to understand that the food we eat is always energized by the impressions we take from our experiences throughout the day. If we have nothing but anger and resentment in the morning, we should wait with cosmic breath as our guide until the good wolf arrives with patience and forgiveness. If we don't, we may feel rushed as if someone is going to take our food from us and we'll rush to consume that anger and resentment, justifying our trauma. Instead, we should feed the good world, and savor each bite as if it's a novel experience on its own as we discover more about ourselves.

Interestingly, we'll often see that even the color of the food has a role to play. Remember the color of emotions exercise we did before? We'll be surprised to know that the colors of emotions manifest in the color of our food, too. For instance, if we have successfully faded any feelings of red to white and to clear, we're ready to eat tomatoes, red bell peppers, and so on. However, if not, then it may so happen that our body rejects the nutrition we receive from it.

Even the linguistic associations we have developed over the years may have a role to play in how we relate to our food. For instance, if we have been overwhelmed with anger, yellow foods might almost seem to signify *yell*-ing; when feeling upset, *grrr*-een may have us growling, while br*own* may turn our frowns around. This may seem almost silly, but we have to know that our subconscious is always at work and finds strange ways of relating to our reality.

The point is we need to recognize when the intuition is being undermined by our racing thoughts, emotional cravings, or feelings of denial. Colors are a playful and measurable way to align with our healing energies. We'll realize that as we discover inspiring ideas, breakthrough emotions, and independent abilities to forgive ourselves for things that went wrong, the manner in which we relate to the water we drink will also change; we'll begin to enjoy the clear water not for any reason but to really enjoy it. This may seem strange to us at first, but the ability to enjoy water is a key indicator that healing is progressing in the right direction.

WATCH WHAT YOU EAT

The idea is to not follow readymade diets, but to find a diet that we relate to physically as well as emotionally. Notice the diet and exercise patterns we currently have. The days that our anxieties come full-fledged are more likely to be the days we've had a sluggish routine.

With regards to diet, we should notice how the colors of the foods we eat may be tied to the emotions and words we used to describe our trauma. As we move through our healing journey, we will automatically start liking different kinds of foods. Be aware of this change.

We may even change our diet proactively by using the musical scale exercise with the color of foods, eventually moving towards the clear in the eye of our mind. Once we've done this, we may realize that we have now started enjoying the foods that were causing digestive problems before. We're now drawing the nutrition we're supposed to from these foods as our body isn't rejecting it on the basis of color association anymore. We have learned how to refuel our body with cosmic breathing. Next, we'll learn to replenish ourselves with soul food and healthy eating.

PART III

CHAPTER 6: REARM YOURSELF

The emotions we discovered and colored are now indications of triumph over insurmountable odds. They were once slivers in our skin, stones in our boots, and trip hazards in our path. But we've purified them with the scale of song notes and digested them fully. We've permitted ourselves to remember our innocence and begun the inward journey for a deeper connection with our core.

Now it's time to invite others into this space and connect outward with our environment in the same innocent, empathetic, and loving manner. A crucial part of taking on this outward journey is establishing healthy boundaries. We might notice that the trauma in our past may have forced us to react in one of two ways—we may either be tempted to shut everyone out or let everyone in. Both extremes can immediately send us back to a place of hurt.

It's time to identify the pattern we engage in when relating to people and the emotions attached to it. The two most frequent emotions that come with these patterns are guilt and shame. Both of these come from a perception of internal inadequacy. The first and the most important thing to remind ourselves is that whatever we have been through was not our fault and that we can heal. Using the musical scale exercise for these feelings can help, too. Even though we may not have identified any guilt or shame feelings being related to our personal traumatic experience *before,* it might be worth a shot to see if guilt and shame are something that we've related to in the *after*math of the trauma, so to speak.

The reason is that this determines our prerequisite for setting healthy boundaries! We will soon realize that a joyous life is about a never-ending back-and-forth between finding our own comfort zone and finding the courage to move out of it, every now and then. So, using boundaries in our everyday affairs will require a constant evaluation between feelings of vulnerability and trust, and not permitting anyone to cross our boundaries before we have checked in with ourselves using these methods. In this way, boundaries form a safe zone in which we nurture our vulnerabilities and only invite someone through when they display nurturing attitudes aligned with our own.

BOUNDARY-SETTING

The first step in establishing healthy boundaries is being aware of our reactions when we engage with people. For instance, when someone approaches us with a request that's impossible for us to fulfill, do we pick a fight or submit to every request no matter how difficult we find it? Do we find it difficult to say 'no' without turning aggressive? If your answer is 'yes,' then try practicing the following statements that we can use when there is a conflict of interest between us and others:

1. "I am not comfortable with that."

2. "I will not be able to fulfill that request."

3. "That doesn't really work for me."

We should write our own statements, using our own words too. The point is to practice saying 'no' in an assertive rather than an aggressive manner.

When ready, we should open up and engage in activities like: exercising with others, eating together, listening to music in a group--so as to have the opportunity to practice healthy boundaries. We should respect the privacy of those around us and make it clear that they should respect ours too by smiling when we feel nurtured and using prepared phrases when not. We should remind people of our boundaries by living them and enforcing them within ourselves in intuitive ways—place a note on the fridge at home or on the locker at work with "Dan's cheese, don't touch" or "Dan's locker for boots & jackets." We should make it lighthearted as we permit others to do the same.

CHAPTER 7: FORGIVE YOURSELF AND OTHERS

There can be no healing without forgiveness. People often find themselves conflicted when it comes to forgiveness because they view it as an external construct with a definite cause-and-effect structure. Only when someone apologizes can we forgive them, is it not so? This myth has forced us to contain all that pain and anger within ourselves for all that time. Forgiveness is an absolutely internal process—it has nothing to do with whether another has asked for it. We forgive because we wish to release ourselves from the negativity that has infected us for so long. Regardless of whether the other person deserves it or not, we forgive because *we* deserve it.

It's not all about forgiving the other person either. Forgiving ourselves is an essential part of forgiving those around us. Sometimes this may be much harder to do than forgiving another person. We have been harsh on ourselves for too long now. It's time to treat ourselves with the same dignity and love that e would treat a friend. We should know in our heart that we deserve equal kindness to what kindness we give others.

The feelings of guilt and shame that we talked about previously, frequently act as a bump in the road to forgiveness—both of ourselves and others. They provoke and worsen our trauma, ultimately turning it into C-PTSD. The act of forgiving ourselves and others starves shame from taking hold of our attention and frees us from its grip. Let's ask for forgiveness from others and give ourselves the time to reach the zone of healing with self-compassion.

Remember, these emotions can be a useful tool to embrace empathy for the suffering of others, too. The only reason anyone experiences shame and guilt is through insecurity. We have already created our security network as we established boundaries and a definitive pathway to healing. Now we can replace the feelings of guilt and shame with a much more positive emotion, like empathy—rather than criticizing ourselves for the mistakes we've made, it might be more helpful to genuinely attempt to understand the impact of these actions on others, to walk in their shoes, and gain a fuller view of their suffering.

WORKING THROUGH SHAME AND GUILT

First and foremost start with this mantra:

"I forgive myself and others for yesterday's events. Today is a new day, and I welcome the opportunity to heal myself as well as others."

We should say this to ourselves every night before we go to bed. It's important, though, that we don't just say it, but also feel the forgiveness running through our body. Feel the freedom that comes with it, as well as the joy that it brings us from knowing we are not tied down by the shackles of pain anymore.

We should simultaneously start releasing shame and guilt, out of our system.

When eating our meal, we can make ourselves two glasses of water—one for ourselves, and one for anything we feel ashamed or guilty about. In our mind, we try to meet the eyes of all those who suffered and wish for their thirst to be quenched, by placing the glass of water on the table, in the fridge, or in a window sill. The next day, we return to the glass of water and pour it in a sink, in a potted plant, or give it away. We are consciously placing those unwanted feelings in this glass every day and letting them go, getting closer to forgiving ourselves completely.

We should repeat this until we have made shame and guilt *allies* of empathy and forgiveness.

CHAPTER 8: APOLOGIZE FREELY

Let's recognize that we have come far from the first moment when we started this journey. We may not have reached the destination yet, but we are certainly on the right path. As we go about engaging in life with these new perspectives and taking risks to heal, remember we should not be too hard on ourselves. It's inevitable that we will trip on this path and relapse into some old, unhealthy patterns sometimes. Our success is not determined by how many times we fall down, but by how well we get up, dust ourselves off, and move on! Yes, we can do this!

Sometimes the innocence of our zone of new perspective will free us of previously adverse circumstances, which originally led us to C-PTSD. But by actively leaving our comfort zone, we're already a step forward towards healing. Let's follow along on our goal to complete the journey and partner with others by giving them our authentic self—the true us. We need to let them know the person we are, even though it may displease them on some occasions.

THE ART OF GENUINE CONNECTIONS

We should try to connect with those around us. We do this by finding people who share a common joy when it comes to making the healing journey. I say, we should invite them into our lives when we are free from guilt and shame. Once we have worked through the shame and guilt, we will be able to look at people in the eyes as equals rather than as superiors or inferiors. When this happens, asking for forgiveness is nothing but a genuine act of connection.

Let's remember that we are asking for forgiveness for actions and behaviors which may have hampered the healing journeys of those around us, not for who we are and how we feel. Once we are clear about this distinction, the apology comes easily because we know that a behavior is not our whole self, and it sure doesn't say anything about us as individuals.

Now that we know others are on our healing path with us, we should feel free to say:

"Forgive me, I have been healing for some time. I apologize if I left you wondering about me. I hope you can support me as I complete my healing journey."

A majority of people will say, "It's okay," or "Of course, I'll support you. Anything you need, I'm here." However, if we have no one we can speak to in this way, we should journal our request for forgiveness, and then just let it go. As I wrote before, some of us haven't found out how to seek forgiveness, but we can certainly do our best now to find it anywhere possible, especially within ourselves.

PART IV

CHAPTER 9: SEAL THE HEALING

As we go through all of the exercises and incorporate the learnings into our being, we should appreciate all that we have grown into. We are no longer the individual who felt overpowered by our trauma, constantly spending tremendous amounts of energy, repressing and hiding the wounds of our past. We have shown the courage to bring those wounds out in the open. Now it's time to tend to those wounds and wear the scars proudly.

Now, we have looked back and assessed the progress we have made. So, it's time to review the trauma words we found in Part I, and prepare ourselves to enter into and experience our healed trauma in a new manner. The loss we have experienced, in whatever form or shape, will always remain as a scar on our memory. The purpose of this book is not to attempt to erase it, but to tend to it, heal from it, and prevent it from bringing our present life to a halt. There is a wealth of untapped knowledge within every trauma—from which we have to find the bright side, the lesson learned, or more so, reveal the full story which we have to *create* through these exercises. The appraisal of many soldiers who lost their legs, people who experienced rape, and adult children of traumatic households is not to lie and tell them no such events could happen in the future, but to renew their personal faith in themselves, to let them know that beautiful opportunities still await them, and that, by following these exercises, the repetitive pattern of acute trauma will be replaced with the bright spirit of life.

A HEALING REVIEW

Let's revisit the exercise we did in Chapter 1 but with a slight difference.

Again, on a new page, using our trauma as the guiding event to motivate us into writing, write a list of words we have that come to mind that exemplify a ***lesson learned*** in our healing journey. For instance, the healing words might be "calm," "relationships," "patience," and so on. We should feel free to choose any healing words we may relate to.

Same as before, let's use a number to measure the intensity of the importance of this word or emotion, and color it accordingly to make it vivid on the page. Finally, utilize the scale of notes to envision the words moving from color to white to clear. Remember these are prayers for others so that they might find these qualities within themselves to take on their own healing journey. Now, we are all truly transformed.

CHAPTER 10: EMBRACE YOUR SEXUALITY

Sex is like air, it's not important unless you aren't getting any.

- John Callahan

How we see ourselves is an important aspect of how we feel as well as how we heal. A self-image is established by taking an inventory of our feelings, which we have been doing through our healing journey. We have looked inward within ourselves and outward at our loved ones. But we still haven't looked at ourselves in the context of our most intimate relationship—with our partner. Whatever our sexual stripe—it should invoke an appreciation for the everyday effects this orientation has on the shaping of our self-image.

We should get to know ourselves on a deeper level by learning what we like and don't like in a chosen partner. This could be a dream partner that we romanticize about meeting one day, or a partner we already have. How we relate to our partner also tells us a lot about how we have experienced trauma.

A healthy sex life blends into the healing strategy of anyone recovering from the effects of C-PTSD. A healthy ritual between partners or couples helps to build confidence in the sexual arena for both of the individuals. Neither should sacrifice their sexual comfort for the other. Aim to take steps of trust and curiosity, so that both can experience true sexual freedom and satisfaction.

TALK IT OUT

We should start a conversation with our partner. Use a pen and paper in a journal, make a vision board with magazine clippings and a bulletin board, or simply talk it out with the other half.

Go ahead and safely explore sexual interests. The best way to do this is to do a body scan for ourselves. Just think about what we like, dislike, or feel ashamed of. This is important when talking to our partner about how we feel appreciated, touched, and loved. We should be honest with someone before getting into bed with them by describing what we want and don't want.

CONCLUSION: BECOME THE NEW YOU!

There we have it—a concise guide to healing the trauma we have experienced for a long time. Though volumes could be written about this topic, it's been made into a brief workbook that we can turn to every now and then. As we finish this, we might be tempted to feel that the work is done, but the truth is finding joy is an ongoing process. Though we have transcended the pain, we're forever growing into the individual we are destined to be. This is an ongoing, lifelong process.

But as we consolidate the learnings from the journey, it is important to know that we are worth every effort we put into it. We should appreciate ourselves for the new version of ourselves that we have unleashed, much like the phoenix that rises from its own ashes. We have taken the trauma and allowed it to make us both strong and vulnerable at the same time. Within this paradox lies the beauty of the human condition.

May we all keep moving forward on our journey of healing and may we always remember that there is only one thing we were ever born to do—we were born to live free!

Healing Your Inner Child From C-PTSD

A Mind-Body-Spirit Approach to Achieving Emotional Control With Authenticity

Dan Hartman

PREFACE:

THE OPPORTUNITY TO HEAL EXISTS IN EVERYONE

The freedom to acquire knowledge comes with the responsibility to use that knowledge.

- Albert Einstein

I have always been professionally driven by the desire to understand what keeps trauma survivors going. Is the "toughening up" they have experienced over time always a good thing for their present self? After a considerable amount of behavioral medicine experience in working with survivors of trauma, I have come to realize that our society's construct of "moving on" isn't always a healthy path to take for the trauma survivor, especially when they're hastily pushed into it. Most of the survivors have been so conditioned to "not appear weak," they seem to have learned that not talking about the trauma is the only approach to defeating it. Many clients that I used to work with would seem quite surprised by the way the traumatic events, which happened years ago, still imprison them. They would be unable to realize, for years on end, how such and such trauma held them back from psychological freedom.

Over the years, I did some intensive work in cognitive behavior therapy (CBT), acceptance and commitment therapy (ACT), and prolonged exposure therapy (PE). Moreover, I found that other therapies like eye movement desensitization and reprocessing (EMDR) and stress inoculation therapy

(SIT) could be prescribed. Various doses of prescription medications in conjunction with the above therapies could be used, too.

But with the onset of the COVID-19 pandemic, our ideas of health and illness, loneliness and togetherness, trauma and healing, have changed drastically. And I desire to empower any individual who seeks alternative care through integrative measures. Individuals and professionals alike can benefit from this book. It's organized concisely to offer relief from specific aspects of trauma. Bring along your courage on this journey because this book is prepared to help anyone accomplish an amazing feat—to heal and recover from childhood traumas.

Childhood experiences have a unique place in our development. The complexities of each generation, as they modernize, change the landscape of these childhood experiences. Thankfully, the science of psychology and psychotherapy have progressed to acclimatize to the changing nature of these personally intimate experiences to help us heal from adverse childhood experiences (ACEs). We now have enough understanding to prevent these ACEs from harming and causing illness in our lives. Inside this short book, we will see practices and therapies to treat ACEs on our own.

The content of this book is founded on the concepts organized by the American Psychological Association (APA). In no way should any of the recommendations or exercises replace professional counseling or therapy, rather the aim is to complement our journey in mental health. By the end of this book, I hope we unlock our true potential to heal and live a joyous, prosperous life.

INTRODUCTION

The construct of adverse childhood experiences (ACEs) has been widely documented in psychological literature. Such experiences are more common than we'd think. Even though it's been years since we experienced it, it still affects the way we process our emotions and relate to those around us. These ACEs manifest subconsciously in everything from dreaming to eating, eventually turning into complex post-traumatic stress disorder (C-PTSD) if left untreated. These ACEs become behaviors that are well conditioned over time and which are very difficult to recognize. This book will help remove the void created by ACEs that we currently carry through our daily life.

ACEs are like a crutch we currently survive with but know better than to abandon. This is because these ACEs have formed into our personality over the years and we currently depend on them to cope with our present realities, no matter how flawed these patterns are. To get rid of them would be transformative and radical. It seems as simple as dropping the crutch and walking normally. This book will take us through a healing journey so that we can do just that—drop the crutch of ACEs and leave our symptoms of C-PTSD behind as we walk forward, healed.

Childhood trauma is terrible pain. It is a daunting task to devote time to recovering from those experiences to achieve personal freedom. Traumas from our childhood range from extreme abuse—physical, emotional, or sexual, or the perpetual feeling of being neglected, or just being a witness to extreme and pervasive violence, abusive language, and such experiences that come from being a part of a dysfunctional household. This abuse may be inflicted by the people we trust like our parents and caregivers or by strangers. Either way, these experiences condition us into having a core belief to the effect "things are never going to be okay," leading to a strong distrust of the world around us and constant fear of abandonment.

Whatever the experiences are, we have learned to develop defenses around our vulnerabilities, just to survive. Our scars and wounds might be different than another person's, with more or fewer actors in the experience. Ultimately, our experiences are substantial to us and could leave us feeling either completely cast aside and alone, or overwhelmed with emotion and unsure of where to even start the healing process. We may be riding a roller coaster of fear, anger, despair, and anxiety and using coping mechanisms like dissociation to handle our day-to-day affairs. A web of lies, deceit, and denial are all landmarks of unresolved emotional trauma resulting from the pain of those memories.

In a nutshell, we've grown up with unmet emotional needs, maybe in part because our parents possibly had unresolved trauma of their own. This generational effect of trauma needs to be addressed as a priority, and that's exactly what we will be doing in this book. Should we relate to this even remotely, then it's time to read on because this book will develop strategies for us to become mindful and grounded. We will find that by the end of this book, we shall be able to at least begin the journey towards the resolution of our childhood trauma.

Healing from childhood trauma requires a balance of tending to the memories of the past while still living in the present. Sometimes the daily tasks like going to the bank or talking with coworkers, parenting or disciplining children, relating to a spouse or loved one, can all feel overwhelming due to stress, shame, or anxiety. In the following short chapters, we will find the tools to tend to our pain and wounds, without additional stress, by following a healing path.

This book will explain C-PTSD and detail the symptoms which are associated with adverse childhood experiences. By understanding the psychology behind C-PTSD, we will better be able to partner with our health care professionals. Any destructive behaviors we have will be replaced by positive strategies which will be enabled through the use of tools like active engagement with others. We will gain a thorough understanding of ourselves, in turn empowering ourselves to make informed choices as we practice releasing our habits of defensive self-protection. This book will teach anyone to use compassion as a healing power within to tackle confusion, shame, and pain. The child within us has been carrying the hurt for too long and, now, it deserves to be loved, nurtured, and rested. It's time to begin this harmonious healing journey.

PART I:

LEARNING ABOUT C-PTSD

CHAPTER 1:
THE DIAGNOSIS

I was often asked this by the families of my clients—how do I know if my loved one has complex post-traumatic stress disorder (C-PTSD)? And how do I make sure their trauma doesn't turn into C-PTSD? It's natural to feel anxious when we hear a seemingly complicated diagnosis like C-PTSD, both for the individual who has been through the traumatic situation as well as their families. It is important to demystify the idea of this diagnosis.

First and foremost, the diagnosis is not something to be ashamed of, and it definitely doesn't mean we are broken. It simply means that the behaviors we found to cope and survive with are reaching their limitations in giving us a fulfilling life. And the good news is that, just as they were found, they can also be unfound and ultimately replaced by a positive mental state and health-promoting behaviors. We'll get right to the roots of self-criticism, emotional suffering, and relationship roadblocks by washing them away through actions we can take with the self-help practices in this book.

The next thing to be aware of is that everyone experiences stress, even extreme stress in some cases, but not everyone develops PTSD or C-PTSD. This is because, as humans, we are fully equipped to process stress. Think of an accident that we may have been in—we got the necessary medical and emotional help from those around us and that was that. Despite being a stressful situation, we don't necessarily wake up with horrible nightmares about it. It is only when the stress is neglected and never processed that it turns into C-PTSD. In the same instance, if we were to have gotten the physical help but never considered the emotional help, it might so happen that every time we see a car similar to ours in color, model, and so on, it triggers an extreme stress response even though the stressful stimuli of the accident has long been removed from our environment.

When stress becomes normal, repetitive, and ultimately chronic, we term it as C-PTSD. Before it gets to be chronic, it is uncomplicated and simple. Uncomplicated stress can be treated to alleviate symptoms like nightmares, flashbacks, irritability, mood changes, and changes in relationships. This treatment is through therapy, medication, or a combination of both. C-PTSD, on the other hand, is caused by multiple traumatic events or by leaving the simple PTSD untreated. C-PTSD is common from abuse or family violence, exposure to war or community violence, and a sudden loss like the death of a loved one. C-PTSD has a higher intensity of the same symptoms but may also be rendered more complicated by the presence of antisocial personality elements like impulsivity, aggression, substance abuse, as well as rage, depression, and panic.

It's crucial to note that a C-PTSD diagnosis is not meant to label anyone into a condition that we are doomed to live with. Much to the contrary, it is to help us find the resolution within ourselves to heal. Ultimately, it's all about refueling and rearming ourselves with a firm belief that we can heal, not just our present adult self but also our inner child who has felt stifled and emotionally malnourished for far too long.

CHAPTER 2:
LIVING WITH C-PTSD

The second question I used to be asked all the time is—what are the effects of living with C-PTSD? What does it mean to have C-PTSD and how does it impact our daily life? I often hear people saying, "But these are only very rare instances when I lose control of my emotions! It doesn't bother me as much on a daily basis, I have it all under control here!" If we relate to this statement, then let me say that C-PTSD is not an outburst that we experience once in a while. In fact, the list of symptoms is so long, I suggest we breathe fluidly and remark on which ones we exhibit by highlighting this page. Preparing ourselves to be healed requires that we partner up with our intuition to do so. Let my words guide us forward and through.

The effects of traumatic stress are considered major environmental challenges placed on an individual's physical and psychological health. This has implications for our ability to cope with life on a day-to-day basis. It is ever-present in our psyche and is silently present in our emotions, relationships, habits, and so on. Like a battery, C-PTSD drains us of our potential. Ultimately, the struggle to cope with life's challenges shouldn't be undermined by the dysregulation or failure to manage our emotional responses. By observing our temperament, we can witness when we experience mood swings and impulses which sometimes will swerve and push us off our desired pathway towards happiness and satisfaction.

Also, to think of C-PTSD in purely emotional terms would be a folly, especially because it has intense consequences for our physical body too. This is because our brain remains in a perpetual state of hyperarousal which leads to a cascade of symptoms, including musculoskeletal pain, hypertension, hyperlipidemia, obesity, and cardiovascular disease. Chemically, C-PTSD is associated with heightened levels of cortisol, a stress hormone, and cytokines, an inflammatory chemical. Another common symptom is migraine headaches. Heart attacks and strokes are more prevalent amongst those of us who suffer from C-PTSD as our blood vessels don't expand as they should.

It is usually this chronic pain in some form or the other that brings out the more emotional, psychological, and behavioral concerns. To battle the chemical imbalances, many of us often turn to substance use and abuse, which not only does damage to the body through negative self-concept but also exacerbates the symptoms of PTSD. These include alcohol, cigarettes, or more psychoactive substances like marijuana, crack, cocaine, and fentanyl. Excessive release of stress hormones produces disrupted circadian rhythm which affects the hypothalamic-pituitary-adrenal (HPA) axis which changes consumption behaviors producing obesity. This may result in Type II diabetes, depression, especially among women, and can cause major upheavals in relationships.

Nightmares are prevalent among those of us suffering from C-PTSD as sleep is associated with an unsafe state of vigilance. Thus, they overload their cortisol with adrenaline and become chronically fatigued. This is the brain's inability to cope with challenging experiences. The mind-body connection is therefore altered into disharmony without a proper circadian rhythm.

We, as individuals, finds ourselves in a vicious cycle of pain which began with internalized childhood trauma and led to physical symptoms, in turn leading to emotional symptoms which eventually feed back into the trauma, making it even more predominant.

Thankfully, this vicious cycle of learned stress responses can all be reversed. The process is a path of self-discovery that will allow us to heal our wounds from childhood trauma. We will become empowered through self-knowledge and awareness and will find self-acceptance to be our greatest ally. We are also not alone. Not only are their others healing from their past, but therapists are prepared to complement the activities in this book with compassionate understanding. Our actions to complete these exercises will reduce our therapy costs and shorten the time of our recovery.

PART II:

RESOLVING C-PTSD

CHAPTER 3:

HEALING STARTS TODAY

The fact that we are reading this tells me we are ready to be healed, and that the journey begins right this moment. It is time we break the terrible cycle of C-PTSD. In this healing journey, we utilize the best and the most prevalent resource we have—the people around us. We take a peek into the various examples and stories of those who have overcome the constant reminders of pain brought on by C-PTSD and are on their way to realizing their true potential. These are real-life cases, but their names have been changed to maintain the confidentiality of the therapeutic process. It's important to empathize with their stories and learn from the actions they took. Therefore, we must sieve out the powerful insights into a total of nine healing points and use them to shape our own story, confidently and fearlessly. Let's begin.

HEALING POINT 1:

SECURITY AND STABILITY

The proven path to calming anxieties and feeling in control begins with security and feeling protected. Remember that this is likely where it all began—not feeling safe in our childhood. While we couldn't do it for ourselves as a child, we certainly have the power to do it now. Let's be survivors and chalk up our experiences and scars as stories to be overcome. We do this by establishing healthy boundaries and recognizing our zones of safety. This refers to anything that makes us realize that we ourselves are reliable, independent adults who can take care of ourselves. This may include having the practical nature of locking our door at night, intelligently going for a brisk walk in the daytime in a safe neighborhood and having the gracious freedom to cook our own meal at home.

Take the example of David, who was spanked and ridiculed as a child in front of his sisters. He was made to feel worthless at home as his father abused him physically and sexually. The result was that David had no men he could truly trust in his life. As an adult, David decided to start his healing journey by getting an apartment with a male roommate who he could trust. He had a private entrance for himself and a shared kitchen to share with his friend. He had plants outside which he would water and tend to while his roommate cared for the cat. Not only was he protecting himself but was also caring for his plants. He found safety for himself away from his father and could tap into self-care habits without being overwhelmed by feelings of shame.

HEALING POINT 2:

RECONCILIATION WITH THE PAST

Recovering from C-PTSD doesn't mean that the trauma has to be locked away, buried under new positive stimuli. Much to the contrary, healing from trauma can only happen when we find new ways to connect to our past rather than forget or ignore it.

Practice remembering the trauma and mourning the loss, in whatever form we have experienced it, to feel resolved and reconciled from old memories. Slowly, comfort levels will return as we gently reprocess all of the things we have lost due to our trauma. Only when the loss is processed and fully mourned can we live in the present and head towards a healed future. Maintaining security and stability through the mourning process is vital to avoid being overcome with emotions.

David started a journal, along with psychotherapy, to write out his feelings every day. After he described his feelings, he would then write out the multiple experiences he had of his father abusing him. He described that the physical abuse started at 4 years old and lasted until he was 11, while the emotional abuse carried on until he moved away at 18. He describes how he lost his sense of innocence, his faith in love and romance, and even his ability to respect himself.

HEALING POINT 3:

REDISCOVERING SELF

Recovery, in the real sense, is experienced when we take our newfound comfort level and begin to rediscover ourselves. We will find ourselves empowered with a new voice as we try to define ourselves beyond the trauma and the fear. As we become aware of the goals we have missed out on while we were trying to survive the trauma of our past, we being to realize life is full of opportunity. This inspires a sense of purpose and empathy—for us, and others!

For instance, David discovered that by turning to his past, he was finally able to put down the burden of his trauma. He realized he had to unpack his experiences, layer by layer, and this revealed some core insecurities he was able to face with self-care routines he identified through the PE therapy. His self-care habits included getting to his job on time to maintain his career goals, participating in yoga classes to remain fit and athletic, and attending music concerts where he could socialize and make friends.

CHAPTER 4:
HANDLING THE SYMPTOMS

While on the journey to recovery, it is not uncommon for people to experience intermittent episodes of extreme anxiety resulting from reliving the trauma. C-PTSD symptoms have three main characteristics—reexperiencing, avoidance, and pervasive feelings of danger.

I am reminded of a client, Suzie—single mother to a 10-year-old daughter. She came to me complaining of physical symptoms of constant migraines, insomnia, and recurring nightmares. Feeling stressed about raising her young daughter, she confessed to holding onto traumas from her childhood and was afraid she wasn't raising her daughter right.

It is common, as in Suzie's case, that before finding security and protection, we'll reexperience old traumas, often relating them to our present perceived inadequacies. Therefore, we either feel undeserving of security and protection or are unable to find it in your current environment because it has too many associations with the traumas. Either way, these are uncomfortable social situations where an individual with C-PTSD feels socially inept. Finding protection and security might require a therapist or even the authorities. Care should be taken to choose a safe environment for the healing to seriously and safely take place.

HEALING POINT 4:

VISUALIZATION

Visualization is a powerful tool in the healing journey. By training ourselves to harness the power of positive visuals, we can find a great deal of comfort even in an anxiety-inducing circumstance. A visualization exercise would typically proceed in the following manner.

Sit where you please—in a chair or on the bed, anywhere that's calm and comfortable—and visualize an ideal home. Is there a yard? A living room? Who lives in the house? Are there any pets? Do friends and family come to visit? We should carefully imagine going about our day and having conversations with people as we enjoy a wonderful meal and laughter in our ideal home.

Try visualizing things in the present, as if we already have all that we wish for. We should do this when we feel the memories of trauma taking hold of us. When we do this, we should remember not to be mechanical in our approach but experience the visuals, complete with the joy they bring us. It is this joy and positivity that will help calm our anxieties.

Suzie lived in a poor neighborhood with a high crime rate and kept reliving her experiences from her youth when her mother wouldn't provide necessary food or clothing. She would steal without telling her mother—clothes and food, just to fulfill her needs as a young girl. Now, as she struggles to pay bills and make ends meet, she frequently found herself reliving her childhood when she felt utterly powerless and insecure. The negative emotions were compounded by her worry that her daughter would engage in the same reckless behavior she engaged in as a child. After she came to see me, we decided that stress inoculation therapy would be best for her where we prepared, in advance, for the triggers and pitfalls she is likely to face in her healing process. She was eventually able to understand her stress responses much better and have routines in place to manage those responses effectively.

Sometimes, however, rather than tackling the stressors head-on, we might be tempted to take the easier way out by avoiding the situations that cause stress. So, rather than getting to our job on time, we skip going to work altogether because of our boss; rather than spending time with family, we avoid them for the fear of getting into another argument. Anxiety of what someone might say or do, which could trigger a stressful event, is ever-present, and we might want to withdraw from activities that other people engage in to limit these stresses. But remember that all this avoidance does is keep us from living a full life. Moreover, running from stressors may not always be helpful as stressors that are out of our control will still pop up, triggering extreme negative emotions due to the lack of preparation.

HEALING POINT 5:

AFFIRMATIONS

A big part of our trauma is that we have never found the reassurance from someone that things will be okay. Affirmations, thus, carry significant value. Turn on some calming music like Beethoven or Mozart, and practice using this positive dialogue sequencing in the mirror:

5. I am okay, I am comfortable, I can handle this.
6. My emotions are important, just like everyone else's.
7. I am joyfully satisfied with myself.

With just these few sentences, we can move one step closer to being prepared for any emotional upheaval. Normalizing our feelings, rather than stigmatizing them, is a big step in recovery. Giving ourselves a break and using a positive attitude to move ahead lets us keep our commitments while honoring those of others, too. Just be wary of taking on too much; there is only so much that can be done in one day, and even when we are on a positive high that makes us feel like we can take on the world, it's wiser to pace ourselves than to run out of steam halfway.

Suzie was emotionally distraught as she described her weekly routine to care for her daughter—it was obvious she was afraid for her daughter's safety and was worried her daughter will take unwarranted risks in theft and criminal behavior in the future. Her trauma was eviscerating her relationship with herself. She doesn't like her distressing memories, thoughts, and feelings. This could have easily escalated into behaviors like refusing to attend therapy, refusing to talk to loved ones, or even pretending the trauma didn't exist. Thankfully, Suzie had the bravery to speak about her trauma.

HEALING POINT 6:

FORGIVENESS AND ACCEPTANCE

Before we even think of forgiving those who inflicted the trauma upon us, we must forgive ourselves. Often, hidden deep underneath the anger, fear, and other such overwhelming emotions is a feeling of deep shame. In Suzie's case, it was the deep shame about her criminal behavior and, at a deeper level, the shame that comes with feeling so helpless. Reminding ourselves that we did the best we could is vital. We need to forgive ourselves to accept shame as a resource for empathy, not a trigger for action. We need to find time to understand that making mistakes is part of life and that perfection is an attitude of practice, not a result we can achieve. Remember that the decisions we made in our childhood were focused on our survival. It's okay to connect with the innocence that was repressed while we fought to cope, the inner child that needs to be nurtured, loved, and cared for.

Suzie would frequently feel disempowered by her relationship with her mother and would return to shame-based behaviors and emotions when the threat of visiting her mother was on the horizon. This threat became an uncontrollable sense of danger as she now kept trying to protect her daughter from her mother's influence.

Now, she holds a boundary that doesn't allow her mother into her house, as she recognizes how she feels triggered by her childhood experience. She has now set the standard of behavior for her mother to live up to. Only if her mother lives up to her commitments and offers behavior Suzie can trust, will her visits to see her granddaughter be permitted. Notice how Suzie uses her shame as a tool to empathize with her mother by not holding a grudge against her and yet establishing firm healthy boundaries. Now, Suzie is sleeping better and doesn't experience frequent headaches. When she analyzes her triggers, Suzie is learning the extent of unfinished business between her and her mother. She takes care to foster a healthy environment for her daughter as a result.

CHAPTER 5:

C-PTSD, DEPRESSION, TOLERANCE

Congratulations! We are forming a relationship with ourselves—the most important relationship of all. As we do this more frequently, our capability to connect with others, using empathy, integrity, and honesty, flourishes. These attributes of our character are what we can faithfully lean on as we begin to handle the next aspect of C-PTSD—depression.

A woman named Mona came to me once with terrible feelings of inadequacy and depression as well as a sore back and neck, which she didn't understand. Responding to how she deals with stress, she replied, "What do you mean? Stress is a given in life, I'm single and it's just me, so I face it every day." Mona is very successful, so I asked further, about whether she experienced stress in her youth. She admitted to playing on furniture as a child and then all of a sudden being put to work at the local restaurant with her mother because her father left, and her mother couldn't afford a babysitter. Her father leaving made her feel unwanted and invalidated as a child which began to manifest as a negative self-image. She was also hypercritical of herself and didn't want to expose her vulnerabilities. In therapy, she learned that her negative self-image was catching up with her and causing her depression. She agreed that she doesn't communicate her needs to anyone as a result of childhood neglect. This acceptance resulted in tremendous breakthroughs and made space for painful emotions of anger and resentment to be released in tears and journaling. Mona regularly attends therapy and enjoys the process of discovering her lost inner child with eye movement desensitization and reprocessing.

HEALING POINT 7:

THE MIND-BODY CONNECTION

The connection between the body and the mind is squarely oriented with somatic psychology. Somatic awareness is found by observing our body as our emotions take shape. We all carry stress in different ways, but we don't have to let it control us. Our body, when allowed to behave with unlimited expression, is marvelous to behold. If we get angry, you might find our fists and jaw clenching. If we feel anxious, maybe there is a tightness in our chest while breathing. Or we might get dizzy, flushed, and clumsy in moments of shame.

Suppressing our emotions can worsen our depression symptoms. Observing our body as we pass through emotions during the day and take note of our habits—both calming and fidgeting, and subtle feelings. At the end of the day, before bed, we should congratulate ourselves for observing these behaviors and decide to keep observing them and refining them so that they flow with the grace of a river. As we become adept at observing the bodily experience that comes with emotions, we will be less likely to be overpowered by them at unexpected moments. Eventually, these somatic exercises become an internal part of ourselves that can be brought consciously at will into yoga classes, sports teams, gymnasiums, and anywhere we can imagine.

Even though I mention these symptoms in this particular order, we might decide to work on them in a different order based on the intensity of the various symptoms for us. I encourage anyone to do it because that to me suggests an active involvement which is more important than anything else.

Mona revealed many times that as an 8-year-old child in her mother's car when her mother was driving, she often feared for her life. On a few occasions, she remembers people yelling and screaming at her mother, honking horns, and her mother hitting a few cars and driving on. She remembers screaming and crying and later swore never to let anyone drive her around ever again. Mona complains of taking Ubers and would rather walk—no one seems to make her feel safe. Her mother simply laughs condescendingly and seems to not be bothered by her lack of awareness on the road.

People who experienced life-threatening events often experience flashbacks which are recurring, unwanted, distressing memories of trauma. This sometimes also results in upsetting dreams or nightmares. These are internal reminders of ACEs that can result in C-PTSD. This can lead to avoidance of external reminders, like specific people, specific places, and specific things. For Mona, it's her mother, her mother's car, and cars in general.

In these cases, when both internal and external reminders become pervasive, we enter into an altered state of consciousness. Sometimes, this features emotional numbness, a defense against our inability to achieve security and protection. In this case, as in the previous one, avoidance has to be replaced by firm and healthy boundary-setting.

HEALING POINT 8:

EMOTIONAL REGULATION

As we proceed with rediscovering ourselves, emotional regulation becomes quite a necessary skill. To do so requires the right tools to reach into the depth of ourselves as we experience what we're capable of. Let's try repeating this mantra silently in our head throughout the day as we pass through points of quiet self-reflection:

"I am unique, I am expressive, I am capable."

The healing process can sometimes feel like it's up against a wall. We may realize that our symptoms persist despite our efforts. It's important not to feel frustrated and instead appreciate the diversity of tools available to us—a fight response as Suzie fought back to keep her abuser at distance, a flight response that David used to remove himself from the situations, and even a freeze response as used by Mona. It's okay to still fall back on these sometimes—we all use them in times of overwhelming emotion. It's also necessary to remember that the patterns we are trying to change have been in place for a long time and are not going to vanish in a matter of weeks or even months. All the heroes in the stories we've discussed kept at it consistently for some time before they started seeing positive change.

HEALING POINT 9:

STRESS TOLERANCE

From time to time, we might find ourselves having difficulty processing intense emotions. In such cases, we need to build our tolerance for self-regulation. Tolerance is our ability to endure subjective conditions. When it comes to stress tolerance, the idea is to formulate a personal consensus for resolution, which manages stress without emotional dysregulation. Stress tolerance means actively engaging in our day-to-day healing journey with only the desire to experience joy and happiness as a result. In other words, it's the belief that we can experience happiness regardless of the negativity around us.

Here's an activity to help with finding joy. Facing the morning sun, we stand with our arms lifted above our head, feeling the solar energy radiate on our palms. Then, we bring that healing energy into our solar plexus—the spot beneath our ribs, right under our sternum. We then feel, with gratitude and appreciation, the energy running through our chest, our heart pumping it out to the rest of our body. I like to practice this frequently for an increasingly better sense of objectivity.

CONCLUSION:

YOUR INNER CHILD IS ALIVE AND WELL

Recovering from C-PTSD is not an event that will suddenly happen to us. As mentioned in the five chapters in this book, the key is to take charge. The aim is to grow gradually, and at our own pace, into the person we have always wanted to become, all the while being aware that what we want to become is also changing every day.

David, Suzie, and Mona have uncovered tools to manage their hopelessness and despair. The latter stages of therapy will continue for David, Suzie, and Mona. They may still experience dissociative symptoms like amnesia pertaining to ACEs altogether, detachment from reality and their own identity, and so on. While reading about this can feel tremendously intimidating, working through these symptoms is often a normal part of the healing journey. When we're ready, choosing a specific traumatic event as a target for healing is the most appropriate path to take with a therapist by our side.

I know I am thankful for the training I received to usher them through the therapies they deserve. I hope to do the same for anyone. In their future, and ours, I see great potential for long-term growth. This includes seeing them, as well as us, master the healing points that I have offered as complements to therapy, and remaining committed to having faith in our inner child as life goes on.

We've been out of touch with our inner child for so long that we've forgotten what innocence feels like. But no matter how long it's been, our inner child is still waiting for us. Reinvigorate that bond and we'll be able to pick up right where we left off. If we are still having difficulty with that, we should spend time with children now and again—it really helps.

When we emulate the children's ability to see unlimited possibilities, we also begin to see ourselves as someone with immeasurable abilities to heal, both ourselves and others. We'll learn to release our triggers from their emotional and impulsive attachments, and genuinely appreciate everyone for doing the best they can to live a fulfilling life. I hope everyone finds innumerable joys of a connected life while continuing to nourish their inner child for as long as they live.

Habits of Love, Daily Self-Care

Achieve Your True Potential And Enjoy The Glory Of Love

Dan Hartman

For My Wife

From the day you walked into my life, you are all that I think about. You are the reason I breathe. You are the stars in my sky. I wouldn't want this any other way. You are the love of my life.

INTRODUCTION

My friend, care for your psyche, know thyself! For once we know ourselves, we may learn how to care for ourselves.

SOCRATES

Look around and notice the tasks that demand our attention right now—students, professionals, or anyone aspiring to anything—we all want and desire many things, but how much do we desire love. It may be that at this very moment we are drowned in chores, trying to honor our commitments, all of which are begging us to do our best, and we are putting off love for another day.

Here now is a moment for us to come together consciously, to remove ourselves from the burdens of "things-we-must-do," and to ask ourselves what we want to do. For instance, these chores and commitments, how many of them are completely fulfilling and gratifying? Bringing absolute joy? And honestly rejuvenating? Many times, many of us may take that quick nap to shut out the groggy feeling, wishing for it to go away. Afternoons turn into evenings, crash-on-the-couch turns into Netflix-and-chill, and our comfort zone turns into another day found living behind the expectation that things are ok.

In the last couple of years, because of the onset of the covid-19 pandemic, I have observed a wave of conversations about mental health—multiple internet pages post slews of advertising about self-care, including tips to emotionally cope during these dire times. Now, with international struggles leading to war and strife, we have been faced with both hysteria and sometimes sound advice on topics of self-care to remedy this uncertainty. Sure, everyone seems to get by under the premise that we take care of ourselves, but what does that really mean? How do we actually care for ourselves?

As a mental health counsellor, I work with clients from a variety of different backgrounds, and one thing I have realized is that self-care is really a personal form of communication we have with ourselves. It's extremely individual and unique to each of us. In fact, no individuals will ever have the same exact inner dialogue with themselves. So, the phenomenon of self-care might mean a day-spa to relax, or a run to clear the mind, but that is only a vague idea. With this book, I shall narrow down what self-care really is for us all.

I often see the concept of self-care largely misunderstood. When I speak to my clients. Many of them seemed to be so caught up in the messaging from the media, mistaking the idea of "taking a break from things" to be self-care. I found that the reason this is thought to be as self-care is that it turns off our minds and removes us from having to be present—so that we don't feel burdened anymore. Is being present actually a tiresome burden? Normally, whatever burden we think that exists gets numbed out as we move into autopilot mode. We need to understand the fundamentally difference between this autopilot mode and self-care. Autopilot disconnects us from the *burden* of thinking about commitments, life, responsibility and risk. Self-care disconnects us from the burden of the burden itself. With the burden relieved, we can form the habit of connecting with ourselves through self-love, thereby allowing for cycles of awakening and self-realization. Both of these together, from self-care to self-love, completely eliminate any and all burdens.

Another self-care myth I frequently encounter in my practice is that self-care is a selfish act for those already well-off, who are laidback, and who generally avoid making tough decisions—especially crisis decisions. Unfortunately, modern culture encourages us to hustle for the award of self-care, such as the next vacation, despite these apparent feelings of jealousy. Why? Well, our life may be a mixture of many commitments, or a minimalists' reprieve of the same. But unless we keep climbing those ladders, corporate or otherwise, one after another, and keep conquering our daily affairs, we risk losing out to someone else who will. And hence, the only option left in front of us is to keep trekking the mountain of success without turning back! Is there any end in sight as to what success combined with self-care is defined as? Unfortunately, achieving success doesn't mean we'll do the self-care stuff later when we retire. What we have to do, is find the impetus to see the opportunity of introducing real self-care habits into our lives, right now, starting this minute. Our health-care providers—those of us who claim to lead by example—are suffering in the six inches between our ears as we too delay and postpone real, genuine self-care habits for tomorrow. The wait is over as this book will take us through the unknown of our worst habits—the ones we don't want to face—and by using daily self-care as a tool, we will find very enjoyable habits of love as a result.

The healthcare systems have come to understand this the hard way, just like everyone else. I witness the intense stress of institutions trying to promote self-care interventions among their employees to prevent burnout. The same institutions that emphasized high-intensity performance and around the clock shifts have had the rug pulled out from under them—promoting emotional well-being instead. It wouldn't be inaccurate to say that self-care, no matter how intense the crisis, is a foundation we need to rely upon no matter how many letters follow our names.

We shall bust more and more such myths as we go along but now that we have a slight idea of what self-care is not, it's now time to deduce what it is. I look at self-care as the intentional and conscious pursuit of all-rounded wellness of self, and this would include strengthening the realms of body, mind, and spirit. Regardless of the goals we set for ourselves, our self-care habits (or lack thereof) will impact us in our professional as well as our personal life. Though the *impact* of these habits may be interchangeable in our personal and professional life, the habit itself could be widely different because love expresses itself and digests differently between these two parts.

Let me explain what I mean with a third example of yet another self-care entanglement of misery. My clients tell me they have been eating healthy, working out, doing everything they can at work, and can't overcome their dissatisfaction with life—living the same aimless routine, day-in, day-out, never deciding to be anyone. This is because of the *vague* nature of self-care that we have been conditioned to have—a definition built on a sandy foundation. Self-care can be, rather should be, specific and goal oriented. Here then—the *stress* of our burdens is not only physical, but also clearly mental and emotional. Our stress from our burdens and commitments is dependent on our frame of mind and our level of maturity to handle them.

Any lack of conscious self-care measures does very little to alleviate our mental and emotional stresses, leaving us overly tired, jaded and bitter. Any results from disingenuous attempts to do self-care in order to reach that next ladder higher are usually short lived and temporary, typically returning us to autopilot mode. In a nutshell, the mold of our small and mediocre life needs to be broken. We all need to labor through individual forms of self-care, unique to each of us, in order to pull together the many parts of our life into harmony.

WHAT THIS BOOK IS AND ISN'T

Through this book I wish to take you on an adventure, a journey that will continue for years to come. I do not wish to run you through a tips-and-activities guide as though that bubble bath was the only destination to better self-care. I hope that this book will do much more than give you ways of caring for yourself; I hope it lets you discover within yourself, the *reasons* for loving yourself. If every day we find the courage to adopt just one new habit of love, we will have 365 more than we had last year. This book will show us how to find the exponential compound effect of such a practice, which will in turn will fill our lives with an abundance of love—love for ourselves and for everyone else too.

With total urgency I plead that we stay together on this journey through the coming chapters as we demystify the all-encompassing terms of self-care through the new formula of habits of love. We will discover the joy we can invite into our daily lives as we discuss the distinct aspects of life and learn how they intersect, leaving *love* as the major lever of opportunity. Be prepared to be rejuvenated, revitalized, reintegrated, and also healed. There isn't any drink-the-cool-aid or quick-fix—just a few prompts and checks to help you either narrow in, and sort things out—when the moment is right each exercise works on the previous one already completed.

I am not giving anyone ready-to-use habits, nor will I deny any questions about specific habits should you want to contact me about them. Usually, in the beginning, clients often ask me what habits to do, but eventually, we all learn to intuit, that is, we learn to trust ourselves. What I will certainly help everyone with is the required mental equipment required to set goals with, and several boosts of confidence to help map out the journey ahead to reach them.

Now, I know what thoughts might be rushing by at this point—this is going to be so much work! Whatever our reaction, we should just feel good about ourselves at this point, and let any cultural conditioning dissolve as we redefine self-care from the root level. We will apply a little bit of science to emotion, which might be tough to swallow at first, but mentally we are a little mechanical, but believe it or not, everything we feel and think results from the current wiring we have in our brains. Our emotions too, although sometimes just spontaneous, have a deep biological and psychological (and therefore scientific) basis.

Moreover, most of our actions can also be traced back to multiple learning theories. Even if something may feel like it's very natural to us, it's likely that we have acquired such a response from individual experiences—experiences that have either nurtured us to thrive or just taught us how to survive. Take, for instance, the learning of a pleasurable musical instrument like the violin. In the beginning, it's almost hell trying to get everything right, but as time goes by, we may sound just as good if not better than the one who is giving the lessons. I have witnessed profound changes in people's lives when self-care routines are adopted when built on a solid foundation. So don't worry, this foundation I am providing will help nurture what is going to be natural to all of us. Our minds may already be coming up with excuses to find ways to resist learning the secret I am prepared to reveal, but trust your gut and leave those thoughts of self-doubt behind you. We are all valued creations and so we deserve to give ourselves the time and effort to be truly loved for our curiosity in deciding to learn about habits of love.

PART I

UNDERSTANDING DAILY HABITS

Here I introduce you to the wonder behind habits and the infinite impact they can have on the sense of fulfillment we can achieve in our daily life. We discuss the components of both healthy and unhealthy daily habits that we seem to be employing sometimes without even realizing it. It's time to rewire any habits which aren't beneficial change them into ones that can truly improve our lives for the better.

1

THE DAILY HABIT BREAKTHROUGH

You don't create your future. You create your daily habits, and they create your future.

RANDY GAGE

Over the years, I have learned one thing about the human condition, and that is that there isn't anything we can't do, no matter our story of origin—where we come from; and our goal in life—where we are headed. I have found some of us may doubt the human potential, but I reassure you that my clients eviscerate doubt in their tales of hope and bravery. I am constantly surprised, and my faith reaffirmed, at the absolute, endless potential we humans carry within us.

I worked with a woman years back—an "absolute mess" as she put it herself. After her divorce her drinking had gone through the roof, she returned to smoking, and let herself go gaining significant weight. Feeling haunted by the prospect of living a life alone, she felt shattered into a million pieces. I have such a vivid recollection of her sitting completely broken in front of me, wondering out loud, over and over again, "How did I get here?" We decided she wasn't at a dead-end, and thankfully pursued some worthwhile therapy with an aim of something better for her.

We worked through her issues persistently for a little over a year, and, neither of us were expecting her traumas to vanish, but our focus remained on tooling up this smart, independent woman so that she could regain her self-confidence and self-worth. At her decision, she concluded her sessions. As a therapist, that was a sign she had decided to become self-sufficient in learning to fulfill and soothe her own psychological needs.

Life went on, I saw other clients, and before I knew it, two years had passed. Then, as I regularly climbed the steps to my office, I was interrupted by her young smiling face, barely recognizable. Three years earlier, she was crippled by hopelessness and self-doubt. Amazing. She looked younger, much happier, fitter, healthier, and most importantly, hopeful of what was yet to come. She said she had decided to turn her life around and she hadn't been sure she had deserved the breakthrough that she found within herself, until she did. And then, wow.

The sense of wonder from this story of my client is deliberate and distinct—the thing that she managed to tap into was not some magic potion, nor a wish granting wand. It was with simple-to-measure, implement and verify, daily habits that she employed with consistency and persistence.

THE LABOR OF FORMING NEW HABITS

Most of our daily lives revolve around daily routines—going to school or work for example. Habits are formulated through routines by their daily repetition until they eventually become automatic. At such a time, like a reflex, we can depend on our habits, as others depend on us, giving our life shape and also depth, otherwise known as character. Certainly we value character, but sometimes the results of our habits might not always be fulfilling—a parking ticket, an illness, divorce. This instigates self-doubt, worry, and anxiety. Maybe we've been chided by someone to take up self-care habits to prevent such unlikelihood. Or we dive-in, getting hard on ourselves, trying to hit self-care goals right away, forgetting what foundation they should be built on. Fortunately, the labor involved in forming the right habits doesn't have to be painstakingly difficult. It's really quite simple, but it does require an effort, which through will and circumstance makes everything possible.

Maybe we are stuck in circumstances watching others enjoy themselves, but we haven't gotten into the game yet. Or, we have gotten so overwhelmed by things that we are up to our eyeballs and suddenly sacrifice our values to change our character. Or even worse, we can't even recognize the habits we have, and we go on letting years pass without ever getting anywhere. There is hope. When our environments nourish positivity in and around the experience of inculcating good habits through self-care routines, we find fulfilment, which when repeated, instills certainty. Certainty not in the external environment, but the internal—that space between our ears.

I was fortunate to become very fond of reading at a young age. Of course, I belong to a generation that didn't have their world shrunk into a screen. A lot of my love for reading was nurtured in me by my parents, through exciting rituals. I remember a book club, where all of us children would gather in one house each week to share stories from books we were reading—with songs, plays, even storytelling. It was a festival, and now it fosters excitement in me every time I find a book in my hands. This was one of my first vivid experiences of habits of love.

Only when we refrain from giving ourselves ultimatums to form new habits will we actually enjoy the process of incorporating them. True magic occurs as we allow our daily habits to unfold and reveal themselves with unique novelty. As we burden our habits with big-picture goals to such and such a degree, or use over-intellectualizations that happen as we like to intellectualize, the intended joy of those habits might be lost along the way, slumping us into the same old routines.

Incorporating the joyful element in our habits seems easier said than done, especially during the difficult times we have witnessed since the beginning of the covid-19 pandemic. The imposed restrictions made it difficult to even function, let alone practice the most effective and productive rituals. However, it is in times like these that self-care assumes utmost importance. Each and every one of us has had an up-close battle with loss—of loved ones, health, finances, or even the basic freedom of movement. The inability to get together with our loved ones, living under the constant fear of a diagnosis, receiving a positive diagnosis, the uncertainty about vaccinations—we have certainly been through a lot over the two years (at the time of writing this book.) It's natural to feel that anxiety hanging over our head. Wars, famines, disasters, even emergencies will always exist, but we are enlightened now with opportunity. We should take heed of what is available to us—our able bodies, our keen minds, and our loving hearts. It's time to keep making a name for ourselves, isn't it?

Sounds pretty basic, right? Feel like a child again and just enjoy things? Well, to assume we have unlocked the key to successful habits only because we believe in the code of positive thinking is not only over-simplified but also a little bit inaccurate. The habit-formation process to achieve our true potential is much more than simply making ourselves feel good. We need to get to the foundation of it all.

WHAT ARE HABITS AFTER ALL?

Since the beginning of time, humans have never really done well with the idea of change. Despite the economic theories that often refer to humans as homo economicus or rational beings that always act in their own self-interest, we have all been known to drop the ball now and again. We can talk about the fulfilling nature of taking the leap of faith with new habits all we want, but I have seen so many of my clients over the years go down that path where they make the grand start, tick all the boxes but get lost somewhere along the way.

A habit may be defined as a behavior that is so ingrained within an individual that it comes to them without even paying conscious attention. But the question is how does a behavior become a habit, and what about the desired result of love and eternal happiness? How do people take one puff of a cigarette one night and one fine day, years later, wake up to realize that they can't get out of bed until they have smoked an entire one?

Decades ago, a psychologist named B. F. Skinner made a breakthrough discovery that looked at habit-formation from the perspective of the consequences of the behavior. One can increase or decrease the likelihood of the occurrence of a specific behavior by means of reward and punishment. Reward a negative behavior and the association is unfortunately reinforced—as a temporary fix, just like a nicotine high. This explains the functioning of the external environment. But what about internal stimuli—this is, any conscious aspect of choice and reasoning. Is it possible to invoke, say, a natural high?

It doesn't take a neurologist to predict that the brain would have a significant role to play in this habit-formation process. Though the brain's role reduces to a minimum once the habit is formed, the cortex is still diligently involved all the way through. Habits have a special value to our functioning because of all the space they free up in our ever-busy brains. Have you ever had the experience where you have taken the familiar path home without consciously paying attention to it? If yes, then you surely have experienced the magic that habits bring with them.

The brain is brilliant at identifying patterns but it identifies the reward and punishment of those patterns quite efficiently too. The interesting part is yet to come, though. The memories of these patterns are then stored in a part of the brain called the basal ganglia. Now, that would be perfectly fine, except this part is the same area of the brain that's involved in emotions. Hence, when we take that early-morning coffee, though there is no one rewarding us externally, our brain immediately associates the caffeine kick and the uplifted mood with coffee which is why over time it likely turns into a habit of emotional response we can't shake off because we love the emotion. We continue to take that cup of joe even though we may realize that it has slowly grown into a double-pump, a triple-triple, with a donut, and the lovely fritter.

This is where the problem lies—the reason we continue with the habit is that the associations formed are essentially stored in a part of the brain that has nothing to do with rational decision-making. While rational decisions happen in the prefrontal cortex, the basal ganglia are in full throttle when it comes to emotion. Think of the initial reward of the cup of coffee—oh-so great! The chemical reward has slowly normalized until it's expected, and yet the original memory justifies the seeking of continued reward—the sugar, the sweet, until we get a little numbed out, like a joke we've heard 100 times before. Like a traumatic event, the thought of not getting a new reward frightens us, and then a trigger of emotion overtakes our rational thinking, and any impulsivity is denied. This is the way of addicts of all kinds.

Why is this important when we are considering our habits? Since our brains are inherently wired to seek dopamine, the hormone of reward, are we doomed to eternally suffer the consequences of any bad habits? Not at all! Our brains are currently wired, and our brains can be re-wired. The current of power running through our bodies is connected from our brain to our instincts through the central nervous system. The plasticity of our brain's makeup enables us to observe habits being formed and reformed as we move and go about our day. Everything we do, from the flinch to the flex, the yawn to the spasm, has to do with mastering ourselves in the use of our daily habits.

THE HABIT OF LOOKING INWARD

It's often said that people everywhere are almost all the same, what differs is their habits. The wisdom of these habits is nothing new—we have seen multiple successful people harness the power of daily self-care habits. Be it Jeff Bezos, Kamala Harris, Elon Musk, or almost any other individual that has achieved success, they all have their routines that they stick to come what may. I have personally known many such people who ensure nothing gets in the way of their routines, not family, not business, not even travel. I have friends who don't check into a hotel unless it has a gym. Some people may think of this as fussy but this is the commitment that it requires if the habit is to truly change our life. And if we have ever doubted even for a moment, whether we have it inside to give such commitment, we should let it go. Deserving success does require that we earn it, but also that we are ready to change who we are to go along with it. So when we commit to looking inward, self-care habits permit more freedom to accept what we're looking for when we truly want it.

Awakening to the knowledge of knowing what we want doesn't come easy—it takes introspection. Despite having heard many motivational speeches and an abundance of success stories of overachievers, people often struggle with the beginning, identifying the bad habits and letting them go, while replacing them with something else--habits of love. Each beginning is as unique as the individual. Perhaps one technique works for the business mogul, but it might not work for the expecting mother.

Looking inward, for many, can be quite an overwhelming task. What it truly means is that there is no one else to blame, no excuses to hide behind, and no complaints to crib about—everything leads right back to the individual. Psychologist Albert Ellis puts it succinctly, "The best years of your life are the ones in which you decide your problems are your own. You do not blame them on your mother, the ecology, or the president. You realize that you control your own destiny." (A-Z Quotes, n.d.) And that is where the real journey begins. No doubt, we will trip and fall and trip again but it's only when we make these mistakes and then muster the strength to reflect on our vulnerability that we can begin to understand what needs to change.

This awakening can be especially difficult not only for the person doing the introspection but also for their loved ones. I used to see this quite often in my practice too—parents desperately trying to keep their children from making the mistakes that they can see from miles away. Recently I had a conversation with my twin sons. They are all grown up now and studying at the University. They have their own life doing what all kids their age do—drinking, partying, socializing, all of it.

As a parent, I cannot begin to express how worried I am that they might get hurt, that they might do something that's not in their best interest. As a parent, I am always going to want to protect them regardless of how old they get. But over the years I have realized that despite my protection, they are going to get hurt every once in a while. They are going to stumble. My job is to always be there when they are trying to get back up. I only have four rules for them while they are away: "don't abuse alcohol, enlighten your minds with education, make a fulfilling career, and call your mother." I trust that while raising them I have instilled within them the values and responsibilities of maturity so I can step back to see them apply this knowledge in their own life experiments.

Inevitably, the majority of us make mistakes from time-to-time, which is really not the end of the world, is it? I believe, in fact, the discovery of our unconscious bad habits is usually found when we are prepared to acknowledge our mistakes. In the process of habit formation, it's important to remind ourselves every now and then that actions have consequences. While some of us may identify our particular pattern of actions and consequences quite quickly, others may not do it until we hit rock bottom. The desperation, frustration, and hopelessness when we hit this rock bottom can feel like it's impossible to change. The choice is ours—stay at rock bottom, get out, or stay blind to bottoming out again. Any change is the direct result of our personally instituted resolve to decide whether or not we are willing to take advantage of what opportunity life presents to us from moment to moment.

WHERE TO BEGIN?

This is the question that quite often delays us from making any solid start on looking within to discover ourselves. What is especially important as we take on the process of forming good habits, is remembering bad habits will be replaced by habits of love. If we don't remember, then it's easy to justify to others and to ourselves that "what I have is good enough," and "anything more is beyond my capacity." So, despite what constructive habits we may already have, love is the additive we need to use to remeasure the reward and consequence puzzle. Let's break down the walls of good enough and conquer the fear-based conditioning that we have a limited capability. Love is the ultimate tool to reinforce our foundations of daily self-care routines because it becomes the skeleton key to unlock our true potential.

We can take stock of our daily routine—I believe that the summation of our life is hidden in the limited number of decisions we make every day. And, with a quantified number of remaining heartbeats left to count in our lives, why not experience life to the fullest every day until our last day? This way, as we decide to build the right daily habits, our complete experience of life will simply unfold into layers upon layers of opportunity. And, life will become immersed with new experiences, our imagination will be full of complete wonder, and our emotions resplendent in harmonious novelty. Which habits are the best to build as we seek authentic fulfilment? Well, those formed on a foundation of love of course.

CHECK

Now we'll examine our foundation. It's our moment to discover the categories of life in which our habits take part. Through this series of checks, we will be able to see which habits serve our purpose and which ones do not. Ultimately, I am going to lead us into managing not only which habits are good and which are not, but also into the formation of new habits, which will be funneled into the fulfillment of love. This might feel like a tennis score right now, but a complete shift in our reality will occur throughout these checks, until we feel awakened and empowered by our sense of self, wishing to adopt self-care attitudes as often as possible. So, feel encouraged to take the time to do these written exercises.

In the coming chapters, I will point to three major categories of distinct habits, namely:

1. **Play:** our leisure habits
2. **Work:** our professional habits
3. **Love:** our love habits

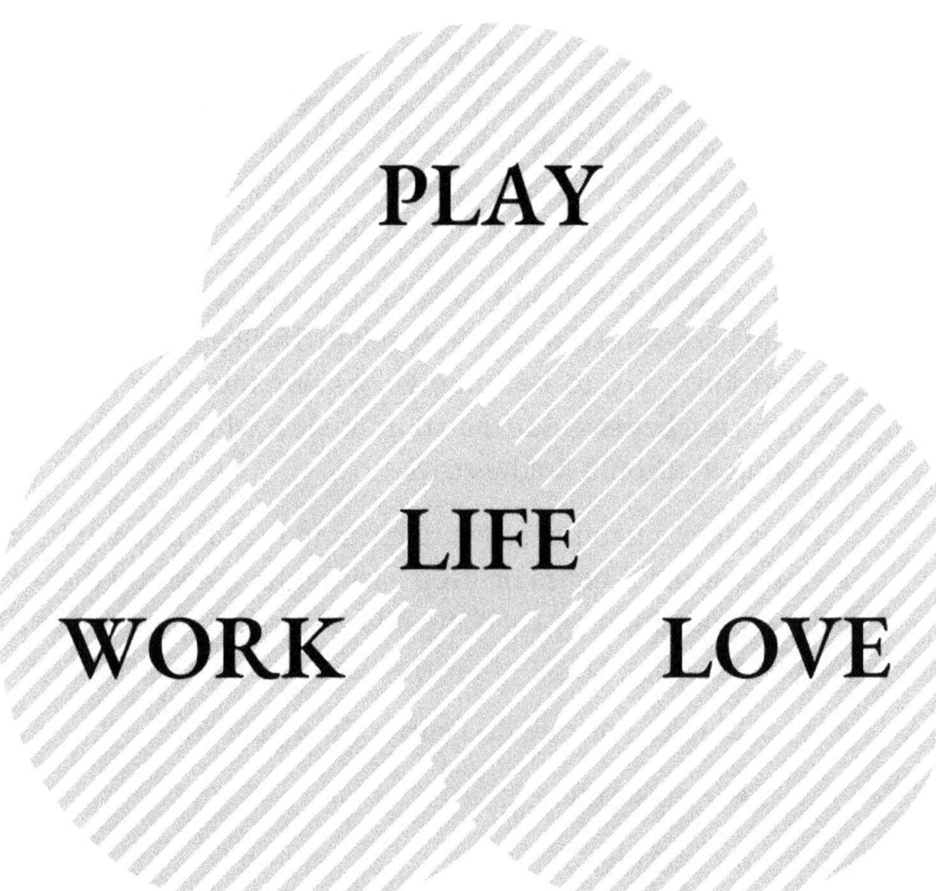

Figure 1. The balanced trifecta of life, with play-work-love

The mixture of activities in life is indeed a multitude. Sometimes people have a balanced split between these three categories in terms of time and energy commitment. But life is very dynamic so this might not always be the case for all of us. The goal of this book is to help us define our life, judge how we would like it to be better, and deliver opportunities for us to do so. The reality is that there may be a certain investment we have already made to each of work, play and love, but I am going to propose how to get a higher return within the limitations of our daily life.

Sit in a quiet place and answer the following questions. Though there is no time limit, try not to dwell on any question for too long. Try to be intuitive, as our intuition, or "gut feeling," is a better guide than our intellect when letting go of anything that could hold us back.

• What does a habit of self-care mean to me? This could be a well-measured 8-hours of sleep each night, a healthy diet of balanced nutrition, or checking into a spiritual retreat once a year.

• What kind of self-care do I currently engage in:

- physically,
- socially,
- emotionally,
- spiritually, and how often?
- This could be a brisk walk with the dog, conversing with colleagues at work, watching the next best blockbuster on Fridays, and attending church once or twice a month.

• What are the top three habits that I would like to develop in the immediate future in each of the three categories—work, play and love? This could be to do things like running 3-miles a day to prepare for that hiking passion me and my spouse both share (for love), getting those concert tickets and listening to the newest album with friends (for play), and finally logging in those hours to the association for a bump in pay (for work).

• How would I like these habits of self-care to benefit me? What's their purpose for me?

• In the next year, can I see myself accomplishing these habits that I have narrowed down?

Remember that when we answer these questions, that the answers are unique and individual to each of us. It's okay to just scratch the surface now because as we go through these pages, we will find more defined ways to go deeper and deeper. Our lives are taking place right now, not tomorrow, nor two weeks from now; so, start with as much honesty as possible. We should be kind to ourselves as we enjoy the process, like a snake shedding its skin, it's completely natural to look at ourselves this way.

Finding purpose with this book and in life, revolves around being honest with what we have a taste for, and grows into what we are ready to try next.

2

INTO THE HABIT LOOP

The truth is you don't break a bad habit, you replace it with a good one.

DENIS WAITLEY

It's a common belief, somehow, that contrary to what Denis Waitley says, we need to break our bad habits. Much like a small child who is being told, constantly, don't play with knives, don't jump on the bed, and don't take candy from a stranger—comprehension is different. The use of negative terms rather than positive ones, to small children, but also to ourselves, results in ineffective habit formation. Come play with this new toy, jump on the mats in the gymnasium, and learn to associate love as a reward instead of candy. You can see, positive encouragement, to anyone, young or old, is opportune and replaces pre-occupation with a inspired vision for something new.

In our upcoming sections, as we dig deeper into the process of changing habits, we should keep paying attention to the opportunities of positive self-communication and assess how it impacts us. We might find these thinking and speaking patterns quite relevant to the habits we wish to change. Regardless of the content of such "don't, don't, don't" self-talk, let's remind ourselves that we can replace these patterns when we acknowledge and accept the harm they are inflicting on ourselves every day—through self-pity, self-denigration, and a lack of self-absolution. The moment that acceptance sets in, the power that these patterns have held over our impulses begins to dissipate, and only when that happens can we begin to make space for new habits and patterns to unleash the best in us.

In the trifecta of life, between work-play-love opportunities, we can therefore see how defining our habits by what we shouldn't do isn't effective. Don't picture a grey elephant standing on a white ball under a red circus tent! Here again, because I have developed a reader's vulnerability to my words, despite using negatives in describing an image, we have all probably visualized it. Therefore, we should be careful to observe what we say and think to ourselves as we follow the routines of our day.

Ultimately, the only way to comprehend the mechanical nature of our mind is to understand the creative energies that fuel the very receptive mental apparatus. Should we want to win at a game, we would need to first decide to play. But by playing, we run the risk of losing. So, we need to first be prepared to lose before the opportunity to win is ever truly available. Preparation precedes opportunity and is realized with an appropriate vision on the screen of our mind. I could project the idea of grey elephants all day like pebbles in your pond, but this book is about love, so we should really get to it. Instead, we can just notice the quality of the temperament required in our mind when instead of a small pebble being dropped into a pond producing little ripples, we have the love of our life in front of us, asking what we want to do next. Without preparation, comprehension cannot spring into action to meet opportunity towards an intended result. But, with the right daily self-care habits, we can certainly love learning how to do it, just like that.

DOWN THE HABIT HOLE

Habits, in general, may seem quite simplistic from the outside—just something we do repeatedly, isn't it? "A settled or regular tendency of practice, especially one that is hard to give up," says the Oxford dictionary (Oxford, 2022). Habits are indeed a result of a prolonged interaction of several cognitive, biological and social factors. From the Journal of American Psychology "[more or less, a fixed way of thinking, willing, or feeling, acquired through previous repetition of mental experience]" (JAP, 2022). And so, our understanding of what we practice and what we settle into are two different things. We may get stimulated into a habit of association, or institute a habit based on attitude and perspective. Either way, both are connected and indeed intertwine, and while survival is the common root, love is ultimately the refined response. At the beginning it might be instinctive, but with practice, it becomes intuitive.

The Cue-Reward Pathway

Whenever I consult with my clients about the science of habit formation, they seem to feel that comprehending this science is in some way equivalent to "cracking the code." While our mechanical nature is indeed a puzzle that when we slowly piece together can reveal new mysteries within ourselves, we should remember that changing habits is not as easy as we might expect. This is a cue to remind ourselves of the organic nature of habit-formation where we learn to become emotionally and mentally prepared for changes to take place in our lives. And believe me, changes do take place. With this understanding, we should leverage our attitudes about love and its underlying subtle force, in order to propel ourselves further ahead on the journey of a successful life experience.

In the 1990s, a team of researchers at MIT did a series of studies that contributed substantially to our present understanding of habits as a whole (Duhigg, 2013.) They learned about how the basal ganglia in the brain is activated through the experience of past memories as well as our present experiences of emotion. A tree of experience is thereby giving fruits to harvest when nurtured.

In his book, *The Power Of Habit* (2013), author Charles Duhigg writes about perceptual theory, defining a cue-routine-reward pathway, offering insight into the practice of human behavior based on his laboratory studies of our biology. Here I break down his theory into three parts.

1. **Cue:** This is what kicks off the habit. Sometimes even referred to as the "reminder", these cues can be virtually anything right from what time of the day it is to a familiar place. For instance, we walk by an alluring hostess inviting us into a cafe. Despite not intending to, we walk right into the cafe and buy a croissant. Most of the time we don't even realize this isn't what we wanted until after we have taken the first bite. And then the guilt takes over. The whole sequence of events is

triggered by the simple smell of baked pastry. Smell is a powerful cue to invoke memory and trigger justification for a routine.

2. **Routine:** This is the actual habit that the cue triggers. Thus, buying the croissant is the routine. The routine might be something being done almost without conscious awareness. Think of the familiar way we go home after school or work—even though we intended to stop at the grocer, we're so familiar with going home, our thinking process had us drive right by the shop. This is to say that there is a certain confidence in the routine act—not getting lost or distracted when going home is a favorable wiring in the brain for a suitable reward. The routine, however, doesn't become automatic all by itself, it still requires the cue. This cue influences the screen of the mind, which is what we are really watching as we rationalize our decision-making processes.

3. **Reward:** This is anything that reinforces a routine. A cheer from the crowd after sinking a basketball shot, or the chemical romance coming from taking another drink. Missed the shot? Perseverance to remember all the hard practice will activate the basal ganglia and drive the emotional desire to try again. Missing intimate connections with others? Here too, the basal ganglia are activated by the habit of drinking. But what sober practice exists for the young and inexperienced lovers to

> draw back upon? Well, let's start with the understanding that the truth of the foundation of every habit relies on the cues of individual desires.

Every cue-routine-reward cycle is a trade-off between fulfillment and hardship, depending on the vision permitted by the foundation established in the individual. You see, what was a good habit in our youth, may no longer serve the same purpose today, or it might still. It depends on the individual's ability to descend into their routine, to analyze it, and refine it. Should the routine already be built on core values of integrity, ethics, and goodwill, refinement processes will be very useful. However, if the routine is indeed cued by reactive, raw, survival instincts from the brain stem, then the temperament of an individual just hasn't evolved from child-rearing days and is still ultimately instinctive. A pouting child may be angry for a mere 20-minutes, while resentment among adults can drive a wedge into a relationship for years and years to come. Thankfully, the emotional maturity of any individual can be refined through daily self-care efforts to find harmony in relationships in order to live freely from such mental ultimatums and silent treatments.

Auto-pilot mode is often a result of individuals still weeping for the care of their parents, like babies would. Instead of realizing what cues exist for a successful habit routine and reward, we return to old, familiar behaviors founded in our childhood, wired into our brains. When childhood habits are founded on trauma, these old habits need to be replaced, as they are likely bad habits, with negative emotions, reinforced by intellectual justifications to survive, "because that's the way we've always done it."

How do we open our hearts to revive our force of love, and terminate those poor thinking patterns and sour moods? We will learn to observe, discern, and decide which habits to keep and improve upon, and which habits to replace, using love as a measurement. Sometimes, individuals like us, without positive family role models, encounter strategies of love founded and modeled on examples which exist in the public eye, through things like movies and books. These might replace a lack of loving encouragement from our never-there-for us-parents, but we still miss the hard truth—that the habits of love we are aiming for always and ultimately originate from parent-child relationships. So, as we reverse engineer Charles Duhigg's cue-routine-reward cycle, we shouldn't neglect the foundation we are standing on. In fact, I've discovered that my clients benefit the most when they find advantage in the habit loop over bad habits learned from childhood.

Breaking the Loop

Once we understand that the cogs and wheels of the habit machine are fixed into position of birth and rebirth, the secrets of positive habit formation begin to reveal themselves most naturally. To avoid crashing, we need to consciously pilot our life successfully. When the screen of the mind is activated by a cue, we should assume control of the yoke and manage our purpose in life with confidence—confidence that our foundation of love will stand strong through the many storms in the sky that Mother Earth requires us to endure.

The foundation of the habit loop is laid in four steps:

1. Routine identification: Examine how often we curse under our breath, feel debased in our thoughts, or blame our significant other for circumstances outside of our control. I know quarrels arrive when children seek to test the capacity they are entitled to when independence is offered by their parents. But, we are adults now, and our entitlement serves no purpose for us. Obviously then, routine identification has its root in our level of established independence from our parents.

2. Reward experimentation: On the promise of love habits being rewarding, we should establish a distinction of when we were betrayed by this expectation, and how. We are betrayed by codependency, which we are generally avoidant to admit, but when it is overcome the habit loop becomes co-generative. This means, as we absorb the fruits of our love habits, our parents can help us to manifest better and better rewards, through no action on their part.

How? Well, reward experimentation is the way, and it is warranted only because it is the basis of the justification for a routine from a cue. I wrote before, perseverance to continue trying basketball shots is good. But under circumstances of repression or abuse from parents (either consciously or unconsciously), many of us won't have resulted in gaining any reward at all—we are left with the memory of practice and survival without any credit. Such emotional trauma conditions our heart to deny and repress positive reward expectations. Instead, we quickly justify our daily life with the examination of commonly expected habits, like going for a run, walking the dog, or taking out the trash. While this might be necessary, habits of love allow us to reach to the root of ultimate fulfillment on a much deeper level. I am not talking about losing a few pounds to look better in the mirror, but shining brightly in the soul, to find an abundance of love for ourselves, to set boundaries on which only equal parts love are accepted. We find out what we desire—unique to ourselves. As easy as this sounds, it's difficult to achieve without using love as a measurement.

3. Trigger isolation: So, we are triggered by the sweet stuff in the coffee? Does it drive us all the way across the city? If our routine is justified by a reward, which it probably is, then at least we are recognizing our independent need to earn credit for our habit loop to function. But, if this trigger is founded on repressed emotions, maligned intentions, ignorant resentments, then unfortunately I conclude it to be a bad habit. Thankfully, these bad habits are worthy of analysis—they can be changed. The change of course happens without sacrificing our need to be nurtured, and we'll pilot the plane of life every day to do so. The way to chart a new path and mark milestones as love-me-knots is created as we recognize cues that align with our aim to achieve our desire.

The cues are sorted into five categories.

1. **Place:** Where am I when I am triggered?
2. **Time:** What time of the day (hour and minute) do I experience the trigger?
3. **Frame of mind:** What course of thoughts are running through my triggered mind?

4. **Audience:** Who else is around me when this trigger begins?
5. **Scene:** What is happening when the trigger is experienced?

It's no mistake that if we measure success by expectations of being loved in return for the love we give, then we will find ourselves betrayed more and more stuck in step 2. Our intuition is the inner pilot of our life, and so, intuitively, we need to handle self-care with the habit of giving more to ourselves and expecting less from others, all the while accepting love as it arrives naturally like rain from the sky. We set the example for our parents, our children, our colleagues, as we root ourselves in the earth on a foundation of truth, while piloting in the air the love-me-nots of daily self-care.

The answers to the above questions and the ensuing self-analysis should be intuitive and not intellectual. To ease into it, many of my clients and I will do simple activities like finger painting, or somatic experiencing. Outside of therapy, this technique of self-questioning is simply termed, self-observation. It's important to give time and energy to actually do this self-observation. And although it does feel like life slows down and we fear we might fall behind in the rat race when we stop to observe ourselves, we are actually taking flight and the "burden" of self-care gets lifted. Our triggers of trauma no longer undermine us, and habits of love result passing us from step 2 to 3.

Implementing change from self-observation requires a mixture of patience and resolve. With enough understanding of what triggers exist in our daily life, we can discern the good from the bad. However, without self-observation, it's clear, no discernment will ever result, and routinely bad habits will continue to be justified. I desired a wife in my young age, and made the habit of envisioning her every day, by journaling and remarking on love I appreciated receiving from my mother and other women. My self-care routine included a really important portion of time in the morning to reflect on my goals as an adult—this was my daily consolidation plan after my self-observation. This plan should also be oriented towards our desires, founded on our birth-right, and unequivocally completed with our understanding of the cue-routine-reward habit loop I described. So, what about love then? Is there a magic, secret cue, that precisely, triggers routines with rewards of love? Yes, and we can discover it.

4. Plan consolidation: let's assemble the instincts I already explained and we already know we have—these are commonly termed the "three" brains—movement, emotion, and intellect. The sexual component to these instincts is the most powerful. This creative force, when left unbridled, is wild and unrefined. To harness it with self-care habits is to handle our creative energies—we do so using our understanding of our desire for sex.

When re-examining ourselves through the five categories of cues, we may realize a cascade of events occurs. When the self-care habit of love is incorporated into the day, we've effectively refined our sexual creative energies and chosen to harness them through merits of the heart. Afterwards, minor triggers no longer affect us the way they did before. This is really a major breakthrough, because we have found the leverage of love to pilot the flight of our life. When the self-care habit of love is ignored, any and all minor triggers are seen to be major disappointments and irritations.

Disappointments leave us in a worm's eye view looking at the world disempowered, as opposed to the bird's eye view, having taken flight. I know what you're thinking, disappointments aren't the end of the world, and it's important to respect the root level work we need to do on this earth as we observe ourselves walking on the ground. And so, just as birds need to descend to the earth to bathe in and drink water, we need to descend into our routines to find triggers that cue us into action. When we become lit up with fire by comprehending our plan of consolidation, we should remember to do so intuitively. This way, as we revisit any daily habits, we will have our individual flight path to follow. Our intuition, or third eye, is our pilot seat, with love as the fuel of our desire.

The Attitudinal Shift

Finding our routine lets us experiment with the reward we enjoy. By analyzing the trigger, we can discern the merit of this enjoyment. And, the plan of consolidation is when we decide to apply new habits for the betterment of our life experience. But, the plan of consolidation really needs to be quite fool-proof. The reason is that the functional core of each habit we currently have is ultimately instinctively sexual. Yes, the basis of any emotional and mental anguish is a result of the ultimate foundation—human sexuality. Summarily, since bad habits are the worst and most difficult to replace, implementing change through them takes an understanding of their dysfunction based on our feelings and thoughts around sex. Getting prepared to act differently to get out of dysfunctional circumstances requires a shift in our attitude and maturity to handle this hot topic. We gain access to the right attitude about sex by learning about the cycle of behavior. I developed this analysis from many years of observation with my clients after seeing them achieve breakthroughs in cognitive behavior therapy (CBT).

In my practice, I often saw people going through more or less four distinct stages when it came to any behavior—desire, will, action, and result. For the purpose of our understanding, let's take a specific behavior we have wanted to change—to improve our love life. Many justifications exist as preparations required ahead of jumping into a relationship with someone new. These are basic tests of character, devoted to evaluating whether or not we are financially prepared, ambitiously oriented, and technically savvy within a refined culture. This is evident in the trifecta of Work/Play/Love goals. A harmony of the three produces a fulfilling cue-

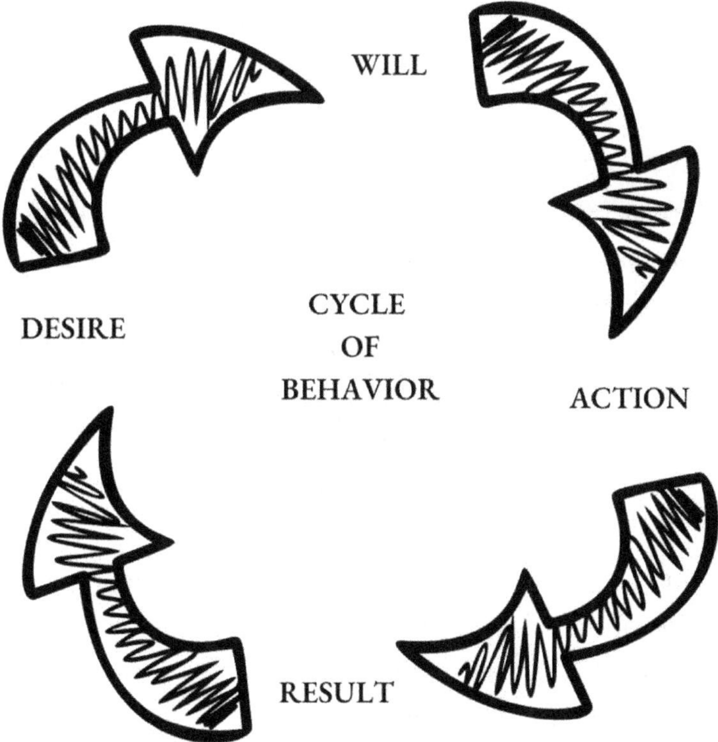

Figure 2. Cycle of behavior: desire, will, action, result

routine-reward series of habits, yet what happens when there isn't enough love? Play? or Work? Disharmony results, and bad habits turn into major problems.

I am certain that the perfect someone is waiting for everyone, and if we carefully pilot our life through the cycle of behavior, we can achieve our dreams of meeting that someone. Or, in the case of renewed faith in an existing marriage, where emotional drama is coming to the forefront, the cycle of behavior, when analyzed and put to practice, will quickly add the necessary depth of empathy and compassion to reformulate and augment the love which was so previously cherished.

Isn't it true that the law of attraction states that when we embody a spirit of abundant joy with radiant love we will attract the same? This is the clue to my second part of the cycle of behavior, that of will, after desire. While the desire to be entangled within the grasps of a passionate lover is usually genuine, the will to act on that desire is sometimes hidden underneath the complexities of intimacy—will they accept me? Am I really attractive? Am I the last piece to their puzzle? Adults are typically familiar with this moment before fantasy becomes reality. It's a moment of evaluation.

It might be useful to be aware that these two stages of desire and will can last for any number of days. I have seen people who seem to be stuck in these two stages throughout their entire lives. So, we should come to realize that the circumstances of evaluating what to do to go from fantasy to reality requires practical measurements and distinct but subtle actions. Fortunately, it's only a matter of knowing that we have the power to take action for us to begin doing it. As such, there isn't any situation without favorable circumstances available to make anyone happy in their quest to find a fulfilling love life.

This book focuses on habits of love, so it's clear now that after the second part, comes the third part—action! And what does action mean? Well, knowing what we want, and taking actions to achieve it will produce a measurable result, however small. A favorable memory, an emotional breakthrough, a crossing of a bridge of trust, sowing seeds of love, committing to marriage, etc. There's no sense in hiding from the course of committing to action, is there? Sexual desire is powerful, and love is apparently blind, so yes, we should also handle these actions with the subtlety they deserve.

Now, any results in the subjective nature of love are always grand and mysterious. In fact, qualitatively, the rich and famous may enjoy the sweet surrender of love, just as the poor and unknown will do the same. What is important between these two cases is that the results coincide with the desires of the individuals. Like a thermometer, sexual desires can be satisfied between people, without ever hitting the hot spots of true intimacy. Lovers generally get better results with patience and practice. To gauge what is important between a couple requires analysis of both quantitative and qualitative results.

We are in the thick of learning to harness the passion of love as a habit. The two dimensions of evaluation (quantity or quality) need to be understood in preparation and in delivery. Obviously, being prepared is essential: knowing what qualities we desire in a spouse will help us judge one when we find one to judge. Again, when faced with commitment, the quantity of emotional investment is sometimes attributed to the practical aspect of moving from fantasy to reality. This might also be a mixture of balancing commitment between work & play, or one's emotional maturity level in intimacy.

We have gone through desire, will, action and result. Now, we return to desire again. A result immediately influences our desire. Now we have a cycle. This first description of the cycle of behavior is modeled on a well-balanced heart—wishing to fulfill a typical romantic pathway of falling in love, getting married and producing offspring. These tangible goals, or milestones, are based on favorable results, given what is typically desired. Not to say this is the only outcome, but when circumstances are going the opposite way, and neither can agree on common goals together, either the relationship with ourselves is failing, or that of us and our lover isn't seeing eye-to-eye.

Taking Advantage of Circumstances

Does the cycle of behavior mean then that we are ultimately at the mercy of the outcomes we achieve? That is, if we receive negative outcomes, are we again doomed? Obviously, no, on both accounts. As anyone who is reading this book can attest, we have free will. Free will, when combined with emotional intelligence, piloted by intuition, allows us to correct the course of our lives from moment-to-moment. With the cycle of behavior, we should note again how many results are both quantitative and qualitative, but so is our perception of the result. This perception is coined as either an advantage or a disadvantage. How so? Well under identical circumstances, two different people will interpret the world in different ways, unique to their desires.

When we evaluate circumstances, we may or may not be led to results which perpetuate opportunities for us to return into the cycle of behavior we enjoy. Our resulting desires and free-will, when left on the table, leaves us with the responsibility to find an advantage in less than favorable circumstances. Luck really has nothing to do with any action we take. This free-market evaluation of desire leading to action is tested by things like: corruption, romance scams, religious conflict, war, etc. To persevere in habits of love through all of that is everything we are looking for.

What many of us don't realize is that it's not receiving an opportunity by sheer luck that makes us successful in our personal pursuits but what we choose to make of those opportunities. I often quote the inspiring rags-to-riches story of the multibillionaire Naveen Jain who owns a unique space program, known as Moonshots and is also a happily married father of two boys. Jain was not born in an affluent household. Much to the contrary, he grew up in one with quite the modest means. And today, he has achieved multiple milestones in the space industry. To put it into perspective, he wasn't offered the opportunities and he would have remained just a face in the crowd if he were to hark on the disadvantages. But with sheer determination, ambition, and hard-work he was able to flip his circumstance to the extent that he has now reached the moon, almost literally.

This may seem idealistic and one-sided, but the lesson here is that when faced with a disadvantageous situation, any one of us has the emotional and cognitive tools to adjust our behaviors, with consistent hard work, all while keeping love as our leverage to achieve desired results. The opposite is sometimes true. Haven't you known someone who feigned affections for so long, on account of this or that? Maybe we did? The advances of a keen lover might be ignored if someone isn't prepared, or if their ego is too proud. There are many reasons of course, but the point is that it's not just the opportunity or lack thereof that matters, but what we choose to do anyway.

The Descending and Ascending Spirals

Realize it or not, we are all making our journeys through similar cycles of behavior simultaneously. Not unlike a pride of lions, all feeding from the same prey, we enjoy such friendly competition. By extension, two broad mindsets should be distinguished because as expected, each of them takes us on a very different daily self-care flight path. The more we understand these, the more we will be able to relate our own attitudes, as well as those of the people around us, to one of these two mindsets. One group believes that life just happens to them, and the other group believes in making choices that can shape the way life turns out. As we do self-observation and we incorporate habits of love, we journey from the former to the latter group.

In the context of our discussion, those of us who view life as a series of failures often find ourselves falling downward into negative habits of resentment, anger, and depression. When we do this, we are always looking for people and things in our surroundings to blame for the negative outcomes in our life. We seem to be perpetually trapped in the cue-trigger-reward habit loop, constantly trying to mentally justify the absence of real pleasure with denial of our abundance of pain.

The guise of keeping a bad habit in the name of the pleasure from mental justification is all too common. This bad habit denies the emotional intelligence derived from facing traumas we all have and healing from them. Psychologists would have us know that Eudaimonism is a fascinating loophole to avoid justifying meanness, arrogance and ego in our establishment of habits of love. Eudaimonism is an understanding of the healing arts, through which pleasure is found from giving life meaning so that we foster emotional intelligence and use it to clean up any pains we might suffer from. Because a heart that seeks meaning beats independently of others, pleasure is indeed a component of desire we should feel to find satisfaction of our individual efforts. Of course, we should do so intuitively. And, we do so with love.

Sometimes, as our mental justifications continue to undermine emotional foundations, we continue to fall prey to negative spirals of thinking, with a strange fear of actually having our emotional needs met. Blinded, we deny credit for deeds we have done well, and continue leading a life others define for us in cue-routine-reward pathways. This might cover up pains of the past that have not yet healed, with temporary pleasures, but having been beaten down, we haven't yet lifted our heads to find dignity. We need to open our eyes to recognize love from the kind hearts who are ready to give it and go after it.

If not, the same spiral has us abandon things that could actually bring us joy, leading to frustrations and ill-behavior towards others and the self. This can be seen in self-destructive and self-sabotaging associations to groups who abuse substances, self-harm, gamble, and so on. These patterns of self-victimization result from negative self-talk on account of unrefined sexual instincts.

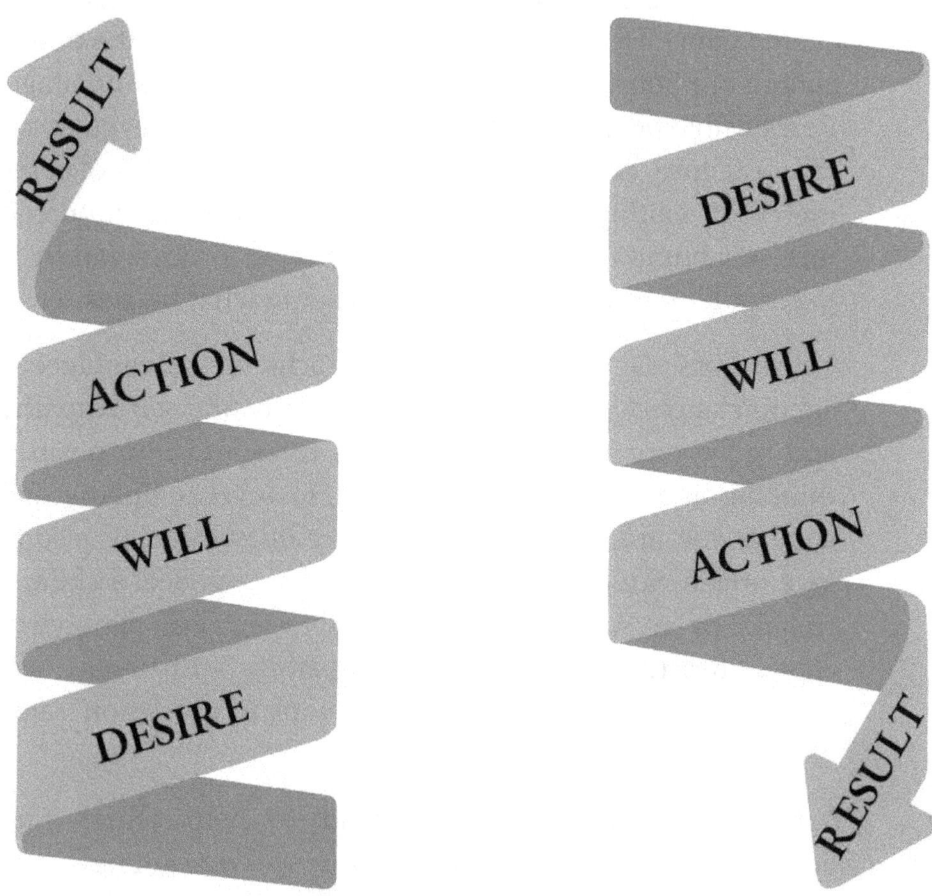

Figure 3. Descending (right) and Ascending (left)

This downward spiral can stop the moment we decide to take responsibility for everything that happens. Of course, taking responsibility is easier said than done and can often be difficult. The moment we take responsibility for ourselves and our lives, we can no longer hide behind the blame and shame game. He or she who is responsible is also the one in charge of piloting their life from disadvantage to advantage. Responsible people make choices and take action even at the risk of failure. Why? Because responsible people are not at the mercy of waiting for a second chance. Some say failure is merely a bump in the road. But, the way to process failure is to consider it as coming one step closer to what we desire.

Those of us who aspire to achieve advantageous circumstances for ourselves will eventually find self-empathy and self-compassion as useful tools to ascend into positive thinking and emotional fulfilment. However, empathy and compassion are not only tools to love ourselves, but also to love others. So, in seeing the plight of a neighbor, a child, a friend, or a lover, we consciously use our emotional capabilities to compassionately empathize with them. This conscious process is known as descending to a common frame of mind.

You see, we consciously descend to help others find advantage in their best capacity. Before we were falling down, and desired to recognize the upward process of fulfilling thoughts and divine emotions. But, instead of giving up hope, blaming and shaming someone for being ill prepared, we provide hands of help, words of wisdom, and hearts burning with fire to inspire cues. The reward of consciously going down through a person's troubles is itself a habit of love. This is experienced by being an example for others to emulate without sacrificing the pleasure of our own rewards. Isn't everyone capable of building habits of love? Tell me, this is a burning question.

Naturally, once capable of consciously descending amongst disadvantageous circumstances to find advantage, anyone can do so virtuously, and repeat it every day. This harvesting of opportunity means that we shouldn't wait for circumstances to present themselves as being favorable—instead, we should originate circumstances for favorable results. This cognitive evaluation means that even when our marriage is on the rocks, it's possible to go one layer deeper, to uncover feelings of fear, misery, or contempt for our spouse, and to realize how these emotions are unfounded, based on naivety or a need to practice forgiveness, asking for it, or giving it.

Now then, when we choose to descend before we ascend, we usually realize we have left our ego outside at the door. Our love habits, simple as they may be, are therefore realized by the powerful tool of deliberate and consistent efforts. A symbiosis is apparent in habits of love between two lovers. When commitment is clear and love is abundantly cherished between two people, they descend for each other intuitively. If this reciprocity doesn't exist, and one is using empathy and compassion to descend while the other is only pre-occupied with ascension, then problems arise. The root of every frame of mind goes unseen and gets missed unless we descend into the emotional realities founded on the basis of sex as a habit of love.

This is why self-care habits are important in practice and preparation. Ultimately, we can master descending to find advantage against all odds for the one we love. This tragedy of unrequited love is long begotten and not forgotten. But we know of the advantage with which we can embrace our innocent birth-right to achieve personal fulfillment at any stage of our life. Young or old, the cycle of behavior is universally enlightening. Its wisdom is essentially a choice to free ourselves from the confines of circumstances that produce a limiting frame of mind. Instead, love becomes the axiom to use before being trigged, and again after as it is its own self-fulfilling reward. This is because the cycle of behavior is used to journey inside ourselves, into our hearts, where it is used to let true love and intimate healing take place.

DOING IT THE SMART WAY

As members of the human race, we are endowed with the unique ability to plan. Our well-developed frontal cortex allows us to imagine what our future would look like. Not only that, but it is also because of this ability to chalk out our life ahead, that we can modulate our current behaviors to reach the vision we have for our futures. It's no secret that goal setting is a major aspect of habit formation. Without a goal to look forward to we are most certainly bound to be lost on our journeys of change even before we begin. And any discussion on goal setting, as you may have guessed, would be incomplete without an understanding of the S.M.A.R.T. technique.

S.M.A.R.T. goal setting has been discussed extensively in the literature on work-life balance and has been zealously propagated in all of the work retreats we have been to. And quite rightly so. S.M.A.R.T. goals are the perfect recipe to track and measure our progress. It's not just the smart acronym though. S.M.A.R.T. stands for Specific, Measurable, Attainable, Relevant, and Time bound. For instance, when someone says, "I want to meet Mr. Right," it's not really a S.M.A.R.T. goal yet because it doesn't state who Mr. Right is, nor when she claims to meet him. Without those criteria, aspirations only remain wishful thinking (fantasy). Earlier on, I made a reference to the in-between of fantasy and reality with respect to desire. Naturally, self-care habits are required to determine within ourselves, how we enjoy our own company first. What S.M.A.R.T. goals will do, when applied to the category of habits of love, is persuade our hearts to be fearless in defining what we really desire.

A S.M.A.R.T. goal technique in the context of our personal life can be both intuitive and glorious. Allow me to explain. My patients say, "This kind of measured approach is all well and good at work with numbers and statistics, but not at home with the spouse and kids!" Such a perspective ignores the fact that we understand how predictability gradually lessens the reward experience. Quantitative goals based on time frames of delivery entice a mixture of desires with the unknown. That is, by offering my spouse the idea of date nights on Fridays, dinner with in-laws on Sundays, vacations, etc, we have a quantity of dates to work with.

If we have nothing to aim for, we won't have a target goal to reach. S.M.A.R.T. goals therefore, in self-care habits, can be assumed to be a test of fulfillment. For instance, my niece went on a date to check if she felt comfortable with this boy's presence. Her milestone came 6 months later, when she told him she loved him. This qualitative breakthrough in maturity was measured with her own courage as she decided to make the lovers leap. Yes, every couple is unique, some in fact are guilty of setting rigid goals, where the point of setting them is lost along the way. We need to tap into setting destinations and enjoying the journey too. Set goals which can be reached, like vacations, thrills rides, weddings, concerts, or even words of commitment. Evaluate their results when the time comes when we expected them to come. The results will help us manage our self-esteem, our self-worth, and our self-image. Goals are really waypoints in our flight to manage our integrity, evaluate our sense of self, and commit again to habits of love. When we value our goals for their purpose to serve our self-care routines, we will want to achieve them. But we should just respect the growth we go through while following that heading.

Let's remark on the fact that we adopt habits not because habits offer us pride in their accomplishment. Gloating of habits we have is also a habit of gloating. Everything is considered in self-observation in so much as the sincerity of realizing what's best for us. The result of successfully adopting self-care habits is only to formulate a life which allows for full self-expression with intimate observation. I've learned that in sharing a new habit or cycle of behavior with someone I trust—I actualize my intention with a resounding self-realization. I got it out of my head, and when I choose to be accountable to myself based on my declaration, what I desire to accomplish actually feels good as I proceed towards it. #habitsoflove

We must be honest. Our society gives us so much in its organization, allowing us to dream at length of what we'd like to do, where we'd like to go, and who we'd like to meet. We have trains, planes, cars; Broadway, Hollywood, Internet; NFL, NBA, MLB; infrastructure, education, fashion, justice, medicine, etc. These establishments were formed by force of desire, will, action and result. This cycle of behavior originated from the five categories of cues, which drove our triggers for routine and reward. Knowing the difference between good and bad habits, allows us to either ascend or descend depending on our comprehension of circumstances. When favorable, we find advantage, when not, it's better to descend consciously to formulate circumstances favorable for an advantage. When these pathways are intuitively felt, it's because we have built our habits of love on a solid foundation. A foundation built on knowing that our relationship with ourselves was given to us by our parents, as well as by our family and peers. We have used measured goals to provide a nurturing sense of reward for a lifetime of growth. And we have confirmed that our partnership with ourselves requires that we recognize work-play-love as definitive aspects of our life which require generous devotion. Let's check and see how this measures up for us.

If you haven't already, now is the time to apply the S.M.A.R.T. goal technique to our love life. Determining what it is we're looking for is going to challenge us to set a marker in the future of when we want to achieve it. And, if our desired outcome is realistic, we'll find ourselves taking actions every day to get closer to the reward of achieving the goal. Our daily self-care check, as we consciously descend to create circumstances favorable to our abilities in getting what we want, will be its own reward. Therefore, not only are we conquering any fears, but we are also triumphing in life. Both are qualities that engender a spirit of resilience and tenacity.

CHECK

Applying the S.M.A.R.T. goal technique to our lives in all three areas—work, play and love—will happen successfully when we decide to consciously adjust and replace any bad habit we have by descending through the cycle of behavior. Where we were once the leading actor in the blame game, we now learn to observe and refrain from such triggers, first becoming an observer of bad routines, then initiating new routines, with new behaviors, and better results. We become the directors, the actors, and the audience in our own lives. Let's take charge and become consciously aware of the rewards which excite and motivate us, as well as the triggers that make us feel helpless. Let's begin by isolating the triggers we commonly face in our everyday life. We should go about this in the following manner:

- Every night before I go to bed, I review the cues, routines, and rewards I observed throughout the day. I note how I felt, what I said, and what I was told.

- Every morning, I make a new plan for events I am expecting to attend to—again, in a journal, or simply on my phone, in my calendar for instance. I could even go so far as to create a VLOG (#habitsoflove) telling anyone what I'm planning on doing, and how I feel about it. What follows here is a simple template to help distinguish the process of incorporating habits of love:

- I analyze the daily/weekly/monthly/yearly pattern to identify triggers and rewards that come

Habit (Good or Bad)	Making the bed Showering Aromatherapy
Time (early or late)	First thing in the morning, 4am Late at night, 9pm Spritz on the pillow, 9:30pm
Reason (this can change)	To sanctify To relax To feel calm
Cues (one or many)	Alarm or spouse Bathroom is available Shopping sale
Results (thoughts, feelings, instincts)	Feels good but hard to do Sometimes rushed Always perfect, I'm oh-so thankful
Consequences (lessons learned)	Feels better having done it Letting others rush me sucks Subtle smell relieves my anxiety with confidence

before and after each habit respectively. However it works out, my reward is measured by my satisfaction in making and achieving my love-goals.

- I reflect upon whether the trigger to an undesirable pattern of behavior is a result of an imbalance in my Work-Life and Play-Life, towards my Love-Life. That is, if I find my love habits are being invaded by too many work goals, perhaps I should evaluate this feeling to see if boundaries are being crossed. For cases when my love habits are overwhelmed by my play goals, perhaps romance isn't there yet, but being friends and socializing shouldn't undermine my self-care habits, which lead to habits of love. It's ok for love-play-work habits to mix, and sometimes this is what I am looking for. I should just be mindful of what's appropriate—work goals can lead to results in love, just as play goals can too. My play-life and work-life might benefit unexpectedly from advances in my love-life.
- Not only is it important to write down and provide reminders to myself of my love goals, but I should track them daily/weekly/monthly/yearly as I pass by the dates I set. I imagine the foundation I can reassure myself with as I become accountable to the desires I hold, year over year. Being flexible to new habits of love is one thing, yes, but also knowing how I function best is living proof that I am reaching my true potential.

New behaviors replacing old behaviors? Good job! Bad habits really do die-hard. But contrary to common belief, old dogs can learn new tricks. We just rely on our foundation, and we will be re-born anew, intuitively. We can trust ourselves to reflect on the influences of our parents in our cycles of behavior, even if they're not 100% perfect memories. This helpful reality often reveals why a harmless smile triggers a bad habit of jealousy and a poor reward of resentment. Such a descending spiral of negative thought and emotion, if left unattended to, could undermine our entire Work-Play-Love trifecta. Children in their innocence, remind us to release those grudges that we cling to so feverishly. Remember that children have love-habits too, and as adults we are honestly very fortunate to raise them and love them altogether.

As we realize the importance of our love-life, we should reflect on how puberty and adulthood influenced our definition of love. Remaining cognizant of this reality allows us to keep our head above water, so we will not lose sight of our individual love goals. As you may remember sex plays a big part in the love goals of others, especially teens.

A harmonious world where everyone experiences love in their own way, is certainly within the vision of this book, wouldn't you agree? Not a single soul should be missed in considerations for the abundance of love that exists constantly all around us. We talked about daily/weekly/monthly/yearly goals, but we could go further, into five-year or ten-year projections. What's important is that we don't change our goals to suit the environment. Remain diligent and observe when we settle for less than we want. Why did we set the goal in the first place? Do we recognize what circumstances we need to have in place to achieve it? Set the goal again. In my experience, the habit of setting goals as high as possible seems defeating until we achieve that first one. Then, a breakthrough occurs, and we will feel gloriously capable of reaching them all. This is the glory of love.

PART II

UNDERSTANDING LOVE

This section explores the link between self-care and habits of love. Self-care is encapsulated by the need to formulate a relationship with ourselves. Once we, ourselves, recognize how our mechanical mind-body-spirit works, we can implore this self-care knowledge and apply it to our desire to love and be loved. Here we look at what love really is and how we have the potential to not only fill our hearts and minds with loving thoughts and actions but recognize and achieve tangible real-world results like a loving family, a loving spouse, and a loving life well lived overall.

3

THE LANGUAGE OF LOVE

Your task is not to seek for love, but merely to seek and find all the barriers within yourself that you have built against it.

RUMI

For centuries, people have tried to put into words this all-engulfing feeling called love. Poets and psychologists alike have attempted to understand what makes love so complicated. Epics and experiments have both talked about what love is, and what it leaves behind. The human race has tried (and continues to try) everything in its power to comprehend the treacherous paths of love and quite frankly, we can only say that love is a mystery we ought to respect.

Evolutionary psychology, as we mentioned before, says that we continue to perform behaviors that help the survival of our species. Would we say that love is one of those behaviors? Interestingly, as many do guess, procreation doesn't require love. Rather, love sometimes exposes us to a risk of heartbreak, where procreation might not. But, after procreation we are left with a child, in which a scene of terrific drama is required to justify our decision to procreate. And once again we return to love as the justification for children, but when it comes to our desire to procreate, we still haven't solved the original heartbreak.

Despite extensive neurological, anthropological, and biological research, we still don't have the answer to this question. So, we are largely left to make our own assumptions about this mysterious thing called love. My assumption goes thus—the reason love has made it through all of humanities evolutions despite issues of corruption, romance scams, and wars is that love lets us thrive. Love hasn't ever been for the faint hearted, only for the brave. Those willing to get out of their comfort zone and explore their feelings and emotions, hopes and dreams, will strive for what they feel they deserve and what they are willing to earn.

There's a certain courage about love, a perpetual persistence, an infinite hope that has made us stick with love despite the heartbreak and pain. Throughout our lives, it's possible to actually understand the metaphor of what it means to "move mountains" for the one we love. How sweet, that the mystery of love continues. And so, myths abound, to teach us of the intuitive love language behind habits of love. The Greek God Zeus, originally found us humans in pairs, with two heads and one body. Fearing our superpowers of sex, he split us in two, cursing us to find the other half again. This yearning and hope is so devised to remind us of the comforting idea of a spiritual soul mate. But further, the gift Zeus offers in his God-like presence, is the memory of a perfect other half, helping us learn how someone yearns for us just as equally as we, them. The nature of this myth is that we can engender a magnetization of loving radiance that we ourselves embody through the courageous process of loving ourselves. Only then, will we reunite with our other half of loving perfection.

SETTING LOVE GOALS

Habits of love are activities that can be done for ourselves, or as a couple. It is not silly to talk about them, although it may tickle the funny bone now and again. Should we have mundane experiences with love, and need to be revitalized or re-invigorated, let ourselves be free to do so. If you are as old as I am, when we used to write love-letters fawning our hearts to crushes, you will know that love goals are always changing and hard to measure. Who writes love letters anymore? I wonder. Naturally, love is like a stone, if left unattended in the shade, it will cool and become cold.

The solution to keeping the stone hot, like the mantle next to the fire, is to use habits of love consistently, with care, and genuine consideration. The elements particular to love are already explained to be both potent and intimate. Therefore, it's really important not to apply too much heat all at once, otherwise emotions might spill over and resentments could arise. Not to justify a lack of will to try, but also to envision a result which is not temporary and without commitment. You see, S.M.A.R.T. love goals intend to imply a measurement of proof which can be shared, touched or experienced along the way.

But when love is applied to S.M.A.R.T. goals, as it should be, subjective elements will always persist. We shouldn't avoid making them objective—how was your date with so-and-so? Did he pop the question yet? Are you dreaming of kids or a home first? Getting out of our head, and into objectivity allows our goals to manifest while still enjoying the dynamic pursuit of favorable results. Those goals, when written down, spoken, or maybe just imagined for now, are the innocent seeds sown to activate an inner discipline to loving ourselves in all past, present and future scenarios.

The best way to break down and understand a habit's course of involvement in our life is to divide it into three phases—initiation, learning, and stability. When this is linked back to the cue-routine-reward pathway we see the multiple dimensions integrated harmoniously. For example, with sufficient desire, we seek to initiate involvement in something interesting, like TikTok, political events, or family birthdays. The habit, which research says, takes about 66 days to form, is only beginning at this point. We have found and initiated an inner discipline to achieve a will for desirable action.

The expense of the second stage is that learning requires all of the following: energy, time, commitment. Beware of absolute attitudes of "all-in" learning. A simple 1% investment gets the ball rolling. We know that if we desire favorable results, we will consciously descend to discover favorable circumstances. Taking action when we find traction under our feet, joy in our step, light-heartedness in our expectations of others, means we may have learned enough to rely on this habit in the next state—that of stability.

Before expecting one habit to produce results on its own, we must understand that life is a constant environment that existed long before we were born and will exist long after we are all gone. So, while a five-minute habit of daily affirmations in the mirror is wise, the benefit of this stable habit will only be realized in the same proportion of our constant daily investment. There is a defined amount of time each day for us to avoid self-sabotage, drop excuses, and make the best of things. When a stable habit is found to reinforce our desires for enlightening thoughts, emotional integrity, and warm heartedness, we have successfully found a useful daily habit to repeat and refine. We can examine this habit as we apply it to the five categories of cues (Place, Time, Frame of Mind, Audience, Scene). How amazing it is to be in control of our ability to experiment safely so that we can live with purpose.

You may have heard of Dr. Arthur Aron's famous 36 Questions that are posed between two strangers. He devised these questions as an experiment to have two complete strangers fall in love. As a psychologist, he and his team conducted the experiment, removing all uncontrolled variables, preparing the strangers to ask these 36 questions, and instructing them to stare into each other's eyes for four minutes after the questions were finished. His intent was to measure closeness and how it affects our hormones, our brain, and our behavior. The results were astounding. Two of the strangers even married shortly thereafter.

Dr. Aron's experiment busts the myth of our subconscious conditioning when it comes to our beliefs about habits of love. Indeed, I do here suggest that any and all couples, or even strangers alike, consensually engage in his love experiment which can be found while searching online. The results we might get for ourselves could be realized quite quickly when we are both seriously intent on moving forward with intimacy and closeness. It expands our predictable routines using a formula that breaks the mold of what we believe to be good enough. Beyond mere traction, these questions are more in the league of propulsion, as if we can suddenly blast into orbit. Now, all that these questions do is really prompt the strangers to gradually reveal aspects about themselves that might actually be increasingly intimate. Questions that only a loving person would generally ask. Our aptitude to enthusiastically experience deeper levels of intimacy definitely requires us to be prepared. You see, none of the following will pass the test: convenient relationships, surface level small talk engagements, and lustful encounters. These pay little heed to getting to know about someone's mother, how they like to be admired, and whether there is empathy for the problems in their life.

I am still quite amazed by the simplicity of Dr. Aron's experiment. It barely allows anyone to really digest the impressions of the other—it lasts about 90 minutes. However, what Dr. Aron has proven is that in his process of descending to find favorable circumstances for both himself and others in the field of study concerning habits of love, is that he has realized a plain and simple pathway to follow. If the shoe fits, wear it. A mark of temptation exists, and it is to expect results from this love pathway without being sincere or authentic with ourselves. We already know, we just need favorable circumstances for ourselves to put our love pathway into effect.

While the results of the love experiment are not wholly ill conceived, they are interestingly worthy of analytical perspectives. Yes, when a couple, even strangers, meet, a mutual desire to complete their will in establishing action for a desired result in habits of love is formed. Then, exponential realizations can occur—people get married, have children, and the mystery of love is proven not to have lost its luster. This romance story shouldn't undermine the unique situation we all face in our life balance of work-play-love, we just need to have faith in it.

CHECK

My wife blushes when I tell her about Dr. Aron's love experiment. I also laugh, you know, it seems too good to be true, doesn't it? It's not, it never was, it's actually always been that way. That story exists every day, all over the place. He and his team simply devised a method to capture it happening live. The cognition required to admit that his experiment could be successful for us, is capable within us. Yes, I truly believe so. I believe in our inner voice, our intuition, the pilot of our third eye, and the way we can achieve our full potential from self-observation, to self-care, and through self-love. Our capacity to love abundantly improves as we love abundantly. With this knowledge, as we carry ourselves throughout our daily affairs, as we watch and observe—old triggers fade away, and new cues are revealed for new routines to begin. Opportunity to overcome past failures, defeats, and rejections will come to us. We should lift our chins, hold our heads high, and remain steadfast in our hearts to manifest the life we want using habits of love. Great things await us.

- I should identify how many questions in Dr. Aron's love experiment I would be comfortable answering and answer them.
- I should reflect on my relationship with the idea of death and the end of life. Do I feel anxious, calm, or humored?
- I should come up with the grandest, most delightful dream of a complete act of self-love I would do for myself. The bigger the better, as no dream is too big for the imagination. With abundant love, I should be capable of realizing my true potential.

4

RADIATING LOVE

We accept the love we think we deserve.

STEPHEN CHBOSKY

Erik Erikson, another celebrated name in psychology, writes about the fact that the experiences a child has with their parents are ultimately crucial throughout their lifespan. He proposes that an individual forms a trusting or a distrusting disposition early in their life based on whether their needs as a child were met consistently. Anyone can explore Erikson's 8-stages of development theory, but here we focus on just the first few. The personality of a child before the age seven is both quite malleable and impressionable and reflects how we are now, after our personality is ultimately formed.

When we start paying attention to our daily patterns and routines, we may be able to notice various degrees of trust in our interactions. Based on stage 1 of Erikson's model, at merely an infant's age, still learning to walk, we would reach for the arms of others, always wanting to be fed and comforted as we pleased. We have obviously learned to discern who to trust with what throughout our day since then—social security numbers and bank passwords shouldn't be passed to strangers! Maybe this was the easy test of our infancy. We have autonomy versus shame, defining will.

As we learned to talk and achieve autonomy—enough to leave the room and come back on our own, we, as children, learned to meet expectations or test boundaries. Healthy realities as a child before the age of 3 involve establishing a will to explore the environment, including the mental environment. Questions get asked, and the inquisitive intellect is formed. Voice interactions are no longer just sounds with tones. As we pass this test against issues of shame, we can realize how Erikson's theory is useful as we remember our ability to recognize parents from strangers, pain from pleasure, and reward and consequence. Now, as adults, if we continually steal, we'd be arrested and shamed under disciplinary laws. A dislike for shame is therefore a useful tool in recognizing how criminal behavior is discouraged. We have initiative versus guilt, defining purpose.

By the age of six or seven, a child has become conscious of themselves, using "I" statements, and can initiate selections from choices based on intellectual reasoning (rational thinking) and emotional reasoning. These are learned behaviors, usually emulated via empathy from their parents. It's satisfactory to write then, that it's possible to teach children to recognize strangers as being something to rationalize in decisions to avoid getting into vans despite prizes of candy or sweets. Such a test of initiative for us should be taught by parents with "don't" instruction but also with positive reinforcement like "do." We don't trust faces we can't recognize but we do enjoy candy and sweets. The test of children trusting what they've learned results in social interactions to feel and measure between industriousness and inferiority, defining competency, self-trust, or confidence.

It is interesting to see how this trust in ourselves translates into how we love and receive love. To have fulfilling relationships, it's essential that we trust more than we mistrust, that we act to reinforce our purpose, and that we competently let people in more than we shut them out. The following is an example of a client whose childhood personality was so vexed that his adult circumstances revealed he needed a significant amount of therapy to heal. Brian was in his late twenties, and he came to me with severe distress about how he hadn't been in even one long-term relationship until then.

When we started talking about his expectations, he revealed some pretty extraordinary ones expressing love through what I could only assume were some enmeshed boundaries. When we talked of other significant women in life, we uncovered that the relationship he shared with his mother was quite abusive in itself, though he didn't realize it at the time. His mother would always keep an excessively close watch on how he spends his time, she would often emotionally blackmail him into spending all his time with her and would frequently make him bail out on his other social engagements, displaying some very confusing and contradictory emotions in a matter of a few minutes, all in the name of his affection.

This was complicated further when Brian started believing that this was love and started expecting the same from his girlfriends. When they didn't reciprocate, he felt almost abandoned and stuck in a loop of negativity. As we progressed with our sessions, I helped him understand how this was leaning closer to emotional abuse than a healthy relationship. He also realized how he was projecting his lack of trust in the relationship with his mother onto all the girlfriends he had had. The fact that he couldn't trust his mother to behave in a consistent and reliable manner was effectively ruining all his adult relationships, even without his knowledge.

He then attended psychotherapy sessions with a colleague of mine who helped him identify the specific triggers and work through them. Though his mother continued to deny unhealthy behaviors on her part, Brian learned to reject this denial and continue with his journey of establishing boundaries of acceptance. Eventually, he found that the problem was not that his partner wouldn't reciprocate but that he was too insecure to let her take the steps towards intimacy from her own place of comfort. Because he was always worried about when the next outburst would be (which is what he was conditioned to by his mother's behavior), he would rather be the one to have an outburst. Once he identified this pattern, he was gradually able to bring this awareness into his present relationship.

The essential point here is that setting love-life goals will require us to use different tools than when we set work-life and play-life goals. When learning habits of love that are new to us, it's important to respect some amount of qualitative easing. That is, take time to absorb the feelings as our brain rewires and we take stock of the intimate changes we've made. Again, we might find that oftentimes we are treading into unknown territory. In this case, we should continue to build self-trust in our self-care routines and know that it's okay to feel immersed in new emotions. As we layer up new emotions within the framework of our existing routines, we experience joy and harmony just as Brian did. However, this can blind us if we aren't fulfilling the balance of giving and receiving love. So, let's use bite-sized progressions, recognize our growth with journaling, vlogs (#habitsoflove), or social media posts, and anchor our milestones with celebrations to recognize those involved in our life.

LOVING THE OTHER

Intellectualizing love is a sure recipe for descending into a spiral of indecision, half-baked ideas, and procrastination. In as much as I myself was a victim of my own childhood only in so much as I let myself be, I too, like Brian, found leverage with self-care habits to process and heal myself into habits of love. Again, I had to get out of my head, as I learned I can't think myself better, nor can I think I am in love. What triggers Brian had to release were those very intimate to him—those from his mother. He had to learn to feel—feel as a child again. He went through bouts of sadness, anger, despair and denial. As he learned what was stolen from him—his innocence and his vulnerability, he realized he was fortunate that he kept his hold onto reality. By reviewing his childhood memories, he descended into his daily routines and discovered multiple triggers with which his abusive mother would manipulate him. Is he at a disadvantage now, without a mother capable of nurturing him? No, he simply had to learn to love the other.

Loving the other is like admiring the city for her organization, the country for her remarkable pride, and mother nature for her abundant bounty of nourishment. Brian found that by forgiving his mother and setting boundaries against previous pains suffered under her bad habits, he gained respect from first himself, but also from others. What is hidden in Brian's example, is my admiration for many men and women wishing to make the leap from a dysfunctional relationship to care better for themselves flying solo.

Narcissists, megalomaniacs, addicts, and the generally abusive other halves will starve us of opportunity and gaslight us into corners of desperation. Our most mighty achievement from these relationships is found in the sober decision to care for ourselves and leave the negative environment. Never is this easy to prescribe nor debate because we usually confide in finding circumstances to our advantage. But, without a rope to tie any love-me-nots, there is no reward to thrive upon. Like a zone of war, therefore, we are left to survive and that's it. You can't push a rope, nor can you pull someone into habits of love they won't recognize, nor practice. Loving the other is a perpetual key of self-respect we enlighten ourselves with. By making choices to prioritize self-care above all else, we can take refuge in the innocence we are afforded in our child-like memories and experiences. We can become single again remembering how our parents conceived and birthed us knowingly. And so that with renewed faith our desire to be loved is warranted, natural, and afforded. Loving the other is a way to preserve our habits of love and nurture our intimacy for the other who deserves it.

Dan Hartman

A Theory of Love

In what ways can we imagine love being important in our life? The word, "love," is sometimes thrown around as a blanket statement denoting positive association to events, places, or things, and typically we recognize it as an important piece of our life puzzle. It's somewhat clear and obvious how we can love a comfortable hat, the sound of a laughing baby, or the feeling of an evening breeze on a hot summer day. However, not all love is the same—I might love my wife equally as much as my mother, but not in the same way. Further, I love my child-self, although it wasn't always this way—I had to learn to remember the positive memories and digest the painful memories as lessons. As my identity changes, so too does the love for myself! As I became a father, there were parts about myself I learned to love more, and other aspects which became less important to me. I love my past-self for who I was, my present-self for who I am, and my future-self for who I will be.

Seeing as our association to the word "love," can be applied, over the course of time, to people, places, and things, we should invite ourselves to examine together what our expectations are in terms of love. We'll do so carefully, with the presentation of a theory. This theory of love I am presenting partners with the also fascinating theory developed by Robert Sternberg. He simplifies the appraisal of the word "love" by triangulating it into three elements, and then further into 7 applicable types. The three elements are: intimacy, passion, and commitment.

When we pick, choose, and combine these elements, individually and together, we develop unique love experiences. It's understood how the complete combination of these three elements gives us the grandest love experience of them all—consummate love. No doubt, unless sparingly applied, or sparsely practiced, consummate love has some predisposed notions of what it is, exactly. And before I define it here in my words, I should write that I only venerate the ideal it represents in relationships, not the judgment of its practice. Let's start with the first relationship and proceed to the last—never mind which is more important than the other.

1. **Liking:** This type of relationship (also known as Intimate Liking) characterizes true friendships. This warm feeling of closeness between two people is like a chemical bond, but not incredibly passionate nor full of commitment for any length of time.

2. **Infatuation:** An infatuation is akin to a "love-at-first-sight" connection, experienced through similar passions. Intimacy and commitment are not necessary, and so infatuation may end suddenly.

3. **Empty love:** This type of love should not be undervalued. Of course, as passion and commitment die, what some people are left with is a love based solely on a commitment of time. Arranged marriages often start in such a manner.

4. **Romantic love:** This is a love that combines intimacy and passion. Here we are not too shy to say that we have combined a liking with arousal. This type of relationship activates sexual hormones in both the man and the woman, and so we have "chemistry."

5. **Fatuous love:** This is a sort of fairytale love which is organized through commitment and passion, with little to no intimacy involved to stabilize or discipline the couple.

6. **Companionate love:** When love is fueled by both intimacy and commitment, we are striking a balance of time spent together with deep connection. Sometimes this is most present with family or as asexual friends.

7. **Consummate love:** By definition, the consummation of a marriage is the act of sexual intercourse. And, in some cultures, this act is quite revered. Therefore, in my eyes, the combination of all of intimacy, passion and commitment should be evaluated wholly before and after any couple ventures into consummate love.

Now, it's probably understood at this point we are reminded that a mother's and father's love is most important when understanding self-care routines, only because those relationships established the foundations of our childhood that we built our adult life on, according to Erikson. The consummate love of our parents, therefore, reveals to us how we can empathize uniquely with them. It also reveals how our immaculate nature is indeed innocent and divine. So, the point of reference for any of us who decide to follow through on our inner calling is always found when independence is therefore reached from our parents.

I mean to write, in a measure of reality, how not only is our return to this innocent place of conception unique, but as fair as fair can be. Even the most desperate son, whose parents exhibit no sign of any of these seven relationship qualities, can still remark on his own grateful inheritance of the earth, as he walks on it, realizing his potential to love. And then even more so, not quite bitten and probably too shy, is the daughter who, despite being born without a home to be nurtured in, can speak to her prayers being answered through Sternberg's consummate love definition. When none of these relationships are given to her, she can still find complete solace in the heart of her divine potential. Qualities that she is so endowed with because of her innate desire to love and be loved.

This makes the comparison of relationships between wife and mother, father and husband, technically complete and thoroughly defined. Yet, where do we go from here with our lives? While staying observant of our desires, careful in our wills, and deliberate in our actions, I hope we are both reaching within to find these understandings to be indelible and indefatigable. Why? Because we are about to double down, to descend even further, now that we know with what ultimate leverage love can be used.

Letting In the Love

The greatest thing you'll ever learn is to love and be loved in return.

NAT KING COLE

The chagrin of all who have fought and lost in the arena of love know very well that what Nat King Cole is saying echoes very strongly in our heart of hearts. Personally, I know it seems like there are few who really vanquish doubt and realize with results who their loved one is. But it is actually all too common. People fall in love, get married, have children, live happily ever after, all the time. Is this the goal in its entirety that all of us are destined to fulfill? If we take another quote, and this time, humbly refresh our sensible work-play-love understanding, we can realize how we are very multidimensional—"Don't confuse our path with our destination." (Quote Fancy, n.d.) This constant reminder illustrates to us the enormous value of refraining from passing judgment on ourselves as we set love-goals.

If our intimacy is losing its footing, we need to descend the spiral of the cycle of behavior to understand the desires we have for the results we want.

If our passion is lacking, we need to descend the spiral of the cycle of behavior to understand the desires we have for the results we want.

If our commitment is losing its integrity, we need to descend the spiral of the cycle of behavior to better understand the desires we have for the result we want.

What I am offering to you in this idea of letting love in, is that until we have purified our desire, it might always be tainted with the expectation of a reward. Naturally, it's clear that certainty is the structure of sanity, so certain rewards are indeed inevitable—the rising sun in the east, the fall of gravity, the wind in our hair. But our intuition is, again, the pilot that flies us through the mystery of love and things of sex. So, let's use it and recognize it.

I have come to know many distinguished gentlemen and ladies as well as talented children, adolescents and young adults. It's not that I found their problems were more or less severe than others who weren't seeking therapy, but that they answered the call within themselves to seek help, find new tools to live with, and adopt better ideas to benefit themselves with. The refusal to become fascinated by the definition of their relationships, and so categorized intellectually, made for a vast number of completely successful healing strategies incorporated. Every one of my patients left using their intuitive abilities to practice love habits in daily self-care routines.

Letting love in therefore, is a peaceful reminder for men to heal any sore spots still triggered through their feminine side. Me, I know, when I descend into behaviors of mine while trying to be a nurturing father, I find powerlessness, and a deep vacancy triggered inside. I describe it like a deep chasm of emotion that I would only hope to tap into if only my children would ask me to.

Women, with their masculine side, round out the comparison of these gender dualities illustrating how empathy functions regardless of gender, but also complimentary to it. Thankfully, women have a masculine side, where creativity originates, gets directed, and emerges. As men learn to be receptive to women, so do women learn independence.

Our willingness to accept who we are in our own hearts, permits us, to whatever the degree, in achieving what we ourselves conceive as our potential. By merits of the heart, therefore, an inner awakening is discovered and finally, we've earned the stripe of ascending to a new habit of love. This love habit may or may not be infused with aromatic aspects of the seven relationships. You could say it would be useful to bring it into the mental massage of analyzing its cues within the 5-categories. But I know for sure, that our hearts will feel lighter, our thoughts free flowing, and emotions harmonized for setting those S.M.A.R.T. love goals.

In the book, A General Theory of Love (2001) by Thomas Lewis, Fari Amini, and Richard Lannon, these three explain how in a relationship, when love is realized as a habit, "one mind revises the other, one heart changes its partner." As psychiatrists, their knowledge of the chemical, neurological processes enlightens us to trust even further how, "the enlightened status as mammals, and neural beings, is limbic revision: the power to remodel the emotional parts of the people we love as our attractors, activates certain limbic pathways, and the brain's inexorable memory pathway remembers them." Lewis aptly says, "Who we are and who we become depends, in part, on whom we love." So, with this added bump of faith from A General Theory of Love, you can feel reassured that just by trying to express ourselves, we are indeed getting somewhere.

"I want a love life, but I don't have one yet," no worries, we've all been there! "I let my love-life diminish," now we know how important it is to us! "I haven't been successful in love yet," admit it, some of us are still learning to be courageous enough to go get it. Normally, desire is found to be a complicated issue. Let me simplify it with you just now. Desire is the intelligence of the heart. Its language is emotion, and it should weigh as much as a feather in your mind.

Hearing Love

You may have seen the image of the three monkeys, who hear no evil, see no evil, and speak no evil. Well, although there are necessary evils in life, my belief is that our ability to purify our heart's desire, is encoded within understanding these three monkeys. I have done this with my patients, as we learn to recognize how love works in our bodies. It really is enjoyable to get into the nitty gritty of being a loving person.

When I listen to the sound of my own heartbeat, I realize my vulnerabilities are the same as those of my neighbor, the criminal, and the policeman. I offer this dichotomy to refrain from judging desire as an innocent emotion. That's why we begin with what love sounds like. Knowing that by vibrating a guitar string in harmony with a resonant frequency, we can inspire emotions that drive delicious thoughts through our mind, and that make us wonder, that's it, just wonder, how a few things might have come to be. There are further studies about sound, not just the sound of a mother's voice reassuring a weeping child, but the voice of a lover, a voice we recognize, a voice we remember, maybe one of tenderness, reassurance, humor, oh, and so much more. The love-music of the sphere of the human condition is a powerful guide to romance the sincerity of our desires. Not only because it inspires the will, but also because when we mark our days by speaking to others the way we want to be spoken to, we've earned merit in our hearts to remain innocent of our need to desire love. Being heard, therefore, is not a requirement of love habits, but speaking our heart is. Should no one be there to listen, find someone who will. To listen and hear is how we recognize, usually with a smile, new results for an action we didn't need to take. When understood, this happiness circumstance is no doubt an advantage for our hearts, because we can do so much with it.

Seeing Love

Love habits in our daily life, should fit together like lock and key. Recognizing ways to see love is going to be found through everyday events in our life. The hardest part about seeing love habits come to fruition is battling the inner desire to feel proud of ourselves. Did I remember to do it? Should I be doing it again? What exactly is it I should be doing? Frankly, our S.M.A.R.T. goals could quite easily fool us into thinking we've accomplished something, when we've only been lying to ourselves. Being accountable to ourselves, with our love goals, is therefore, a very unique challenge.

First, we need to learn to enjoy seeing things as they are, unchanged. Despite what we may not agree with in our minds, we can find a way to agree with it in our hearts. Such a will to choose love over any other motivation is not weak, nor ill advised, but strategic. Yes, it's very intelligent to do so. The reason we need to see things as they are, instead of trying to manipulate things to be like we desire them to be, is because our ultimate power to feel love is found from our acceptance. Acceptance is independence in disguise, and is always mirrored through others, in conflict and in joy. The more independent I am, the more I empower others to be the same.

When we find the nobility to see others experiencing love themselves, however faint, we've let jealousy go and found common ground for friends among enemies. I know that my youngest son used to come up to me and explain how he wanted as many chocolate pancakes as his older brothers, even though he wouldn't eat them. The way he saw the world at breakfast, was to agree with the joy his brothers were experiencing, even though he wasn't eating it. He taught me to see love as a scene to get into. An act to engage in. I was convinced by the way he wanted to be seen in the world, as a loving person, through the influences of his family.

How we see the world will determine how we fit as actors in the scenes from day to day. So, how are we to judge our best behaviors then? We have all of the freedom to behave as we wish, yet, what is the perfect combination of words, emotions, and actions to obtain loving fulfillment? Here is the strategy: by presenting to the world how we see things the way we want them to be, we employ opportunity amongst others. It's therefore a job of the heart to spring our life into action. Do you remember my youngest son? The oft quoted "children should be seen and not heard," has its shortcomings that we can artfully learn to interpret otherwise. Learning to be seen in a desirable way, children first mark their experiences of the world by emulating our words and emotional expressions until finding their own voice and personality. When adults begin seeing love as the discipline of daily acts within the scenes of morning, afternoon, and night, we are at the mercy of evaluation by others until we learn to convince and persuade. The memory of whether we loved enough, is for sure a subjective notion in our hearts. We say to ourselves, "Did the words they heard sink in?" And, "Did I actually take the time to empathize and descend into their life, walking in their shoes?" Love is, therefore, realized as the greatest tool for anyone to move from less opportunity to more—with a simple change of heart. This less is more scenario just simply arrives. Like an instrument of intuition, when we listen to it, it's apparent that when we have loved to our fullest capacity, we will find innocence in our actions. This is known by such words as, "I am," "I was," and "I do." To see the habits of love we've created and been practicing become complete scenes of our own realization is really exciting to experience and enjoy. Again, I return to remind us that these moments of celebration can be missed depending on our perspective and our will to discover the way to a complete life-film. Many marriages end for reasons couples justify within the scene of their life. Other marriages extend to multiple generations, where grandparents enjoy these secrets of innocence.

Feeling Love

As an adolescent, I made many memories learning to live through the parables of adults. I was told as a child, and now I tell my kids,

"You'll be amazed at what you attract after you start to believe in what you deserve."

(LOVE EXPANDS, 2020)

As an adult, I enjoy these sweet sayings as they enlighten the youth of today to think on their own and to both recognize what they like and dislike. Feeling love is not only hanky-panky, but also a soul resounding feeling of tenderness combined with the will to protect vulnerabilities. The intimate look of love from a tender lover, the vulnerable feeling of forever from a lifelong spouse, and the bubbly joy from a smiling child—they all give waves of energy, stemming from hormones like Oxytocin. The institution of resolve to devote a habit to exploring our desire in enjoying these moments is like building a chamber deep inside our heart where we can keep these treasures for our whole life. Yes, this includes rom-coms, romance novels, celebrity crushes, and godly devotions to cultural idealisms. I mean to say, our gut feelings come with a capacity to fight against being too tired to say those kind words, too lazy to read that bedtime story, or too arrogant to admit we want to share our bed with someone. Such feelings shouldn't dismiss, deny, or absolve anyone from taking action, but first, they need to be recognized, wholly felt, and understood, from a place of genuine self-care, self-love, and self-respect.

Feeling love is a practice much akin to checking the weather and is not so much different than self-observation. One particular aspect of feeling love is found in sharing space with others. Cohabitating is a very measured test of our ability to get down and avoid the shallow expectations of the idea of perfection. Being forgiving of differences others share while under the same roof is not so ominous a task if we're prepared with self-care habits as a foundation. Again, don't get me wrong, exclamations of perfection that come from shining moments of eureka are very very welcome. Naturally, we need to learn to listen intently, and see clearly, but also feel lovingly. The heat and potency of this loving feeling becomes more refined as we act with integrity using our powerful, passionate abilities to seize the day, every day.

If no self-care habits are forged in the arena of our daily life, then any attempt to jump into a relationship where we know we need to hear love, see love, and feel love to actually enjoy it, will be undermined by the pressure of showing up to deliver such results. When a couple feels like they have to perform in order to please the other, or else suffer certain consequences, we have a problem! Such pitfalls shouldn't scare us, though, as they are ultimately inevitable. So, by remembering to refrain from that argument, calm that raised voice, and ease the trigger of expectation, we've succeeded in finding the intuition in our heart's desire, which isn't always a direct result of hard work. Maybe a lot of effort, but actually no hard work. The answers we seek to maintain passion, intimacy, and commitment come down to building them up on a foundation that is solid, which will hold up to any dramatical storm the future may throw at us.

Don't get me wrong, hard work is definitely an aspect of every person's life, especially as people of sports, trades, or anyone working through physical therapy can attest; however, the act of seeing, feeling and hearing love, is an inner process, which has little to nothing to do with muscles and bones. Or does it? Well, indirectly it does. What is intricately connected to our body, are the symbiotic pathways of neurokinetic memories originating in the cerebellum. Do you flinch at the sound of thunder? Leap at the sight of spiders? Or salivate at the smell of a burger?

In fact, as we mix certain self-care rituals into our love-life, our instincts will come into the mix again. Maybe we're learning to relax a little more, do some meditation in a group, or experience some light pillow talk. If ever we start falling asleep after tremendous self-observation and meditation, we might even experience a hypnic jerk—a sort of sensation between being asleep and being awake, when we might feel a sudden jolt to disrupt the process of 'falling.' Because habits of love involve re-programming our emotions, the screen of our mind as we relax and dream is going to reveal some very new fantastic imagery and revealing dreams. So, these hypnics are quite normal.

CHECK

Before we go out into the world and conduct our own love experiments, it is necessary to clarify for ourselves what love means to us. How is it that we express our love? How would we like our loved ones to express their love to us? It is important to reflect on these questions to break out of the unproductive loop of assumptions and unsaid expectations.

- When it comes to my partner and I (fantasy or reality), I like to assess the aspects that my relationship has the most of in: passion, intimacy, or commitment. How would I like to bring any missing aspects into the relationship? I should list three activities that I think would help.
- When overcome with emotion, I try to focus on what I am feeling rather than investigating what caused it. If the emotion is jealousy, for instance, I try to become aware of where in my body I feel that jealousy. When I locate the spot, I pay attention to what the emotion is doing to me. If I feel it in my shoulders, for instance, I simply feel the tightness and as I breathe deeply, releasing the jealousy by abiding in the comfort of my breathing. I continue this for as long as I need to feel calm.

PART III

BUILDING HABITS OF LOVE

We are ready to take flight! We've done our series of checks, which means the dream of fulfilling our personal ambition to love and beloved is now ready to be a part of our life. This is both exciting and unnerving because with each step we take, we are moving closer to our goals. Confidence is our motto and love is the way. Aren't you glad we've learned how our cycle of behavior is just mechanical, and yet we can harness our conscious will with our intuition piloting our desires? Let's welcome love and joy into our lives so that we may transform ourselves in the most unexpected ways.

5

LOVE YOURSELF

Love yourself first and everything else falls into line. You really have to love yourself to get anything done in this world.

LUCILLE BALL

From the day we arrive on this earth, we begin to build a life that we will carry with ourselves until the very end. As we grow older this life becomes as much about our social, intellectual, and emotional needs as our physical survival needs, sometimes even more so. The interactive world that we are introduced to when our parents, and family smile at us the first time they hold us, the way they play peekaboo with us, is the first step in learning the value of these interactions. The small baby that cries when the mother leaves the room has begun to understand the lifelong effect that these social interactions will have on us. Growing older in the midst of the social interactions, sometimes positive and sometimes negative, leaves us either content and confident or unfulfilled and unloved. Either way, we find ourselves tangled in the web of love and relationships as they come to define our very existence.

When all our lives we have spent our efforts in receiving the love from others, the idea of self-love can seem almost rebellious, almost as if it's taking us away from the others, almost as if somehow self-love is selfish. The truth is, however, far from this assumption. Self-love is the prerequisite to any form of love that we have talked about till now. Self-love is like the reserve from which we attempt to draw the love we give others. It's only when we love ourselves that we will ever be able to appreciate the true love that someone else showers upon us. In the absence of self-love, however, it's easy to get lost in treacherous paths of love, mistaking even abuse to be love of some kind. It is only when we love ourselves will we be able to see when others are treating us wrongly and will have the courage to say no to exploitative behaviors.

Remembering to love ourselves first is not always easy especially when faced with years of putting ourselves after everything else. But be assured that the decision to love ourselves is a good one, and although we might fall into old habits, these temporary lapses in judgment are certainly forgivable. While we move forward on the path of forming the habit to love ourselves, it's necessary to keep unrealistic expectations at bay. Most of the time, it is these overly rigid and imaginary expectations that make people give up on their habit-formation journeys the moment they experience a setback. They often expect patterns that are years old to vanish in a matter of a few days.

As we tread the ups and downs of the habit-formation process, it's essential to treat ourselves with patience and kindness. Give yourself a chance and appreciate the knowledge that it's possible to remove old habits and replace them with new ones. We no longer depend on others to experience love—why would we when we are the life spring of that love ourselves? Once we uncover this love within, the love we experience from others, from our significant other, our family, and our friends, is only an extension of our own love. And it is when these two forms of love become aligned with each other, that we realize our true potential to love and beloved.

What I find the most interesting is also the manner in which we can manifest this love towards ourselves. One might think this grand form of love would require just the same amount of grandiosity in terms of action. The reality, however, is that we can invite self-love in our life with the simplest of actions. This might start with cleaning our room or making our bed every day, writing notes to ourselves of our greatest dreams, starting a vision board and leaving it open to new ideas every day, and showing loved ones we are taking care of ourselves with "me-time."

THE ACT OF SELF-LOVE

Many years ago, a psychologist named Carl Rogers in his theory on self-concept talked about how we look at ourselves, the value that we place upon ourselves, and the constant struggle to meet the ideal self. It turns out his theory applies very well even today, as we try to explore who we are. Psychologists generally agree that others play a role in developing our self-concept. This means, how we see ourselves comes from how others see us, especially in our formative years. For instance, when a child with encouraging, loving parents grows up to be a confident risk-taker, we commonly attribute this to well modeled behaviors learned in their youth. Similarly, a child with restrictive and over-protective parents would likely grow up with feelings of inadequacy. Framed with this self-concept, usually the second child in this example, would find the burden of self-care quite heavy, resulting in difficulty in their work-play-love relationships.

The point I am making here is that anyone who is embarking on this self-care path towards habits of love, will have their own plane of thoughts/emotions/desires to contend with, and their own intuitive nature to pilot. As such, we cannot do the self-care of someone else, as hard as we try to. Instead, we can illuminate the idea to others, by instituting independence within our very presence. This is unfortunately sometimes judged as selfish, self-righteous, and egotistical. We should pay no heed to such untethered desires, unwarranted judgments, and unrelenting jealousy. Instead, we find empathy and become cognizant of our self-concept. When others walk all over us, set boundaries. When our desires are dismissed and ignored, find others who are receptive. Again, as we observe ourselves we explore our self-concept—many accept victimization unwittingly, while others are bullies to the nth degree. Where do we stand? A healthy self-concept includes mutual respect from others, open communication pathways for individual expression, and regard for discipline and justice against abuse and mistreatment.

Culturally, roles are traditionally assigned between males and females, elders and youth, professional and lay people. These assignments have been evolving—evolving as a result of self-care habits. The reason for the success of self-care habits? Why, they are built on a foundation of love of course. How else would anyone feel convinced to change their ways unless they see that their life benefits. The ability to persuade, convince and enroll others into behavior cycles of success therefore requires definitive knowledge of our concept of self.

Although we cannot do self-care for anyone except for ourselves, we can impress upon others in a way to assist in the matter for them. My wife and I met on the dance floor, and although I wasn't a tremendous dancer, it was through movement that her and I made our first advances. Her impression of me and my impression on her resulted in a wordless few minutes of smiles and gestures. If I or her were too preoccupied with work-life and play-life, we would have interpreted those impressions differently. A soft touch, a patient heart, and a sincere tone of voice all help to transform the impressions another person is receiving from the outside world. Clearly what this means is, I encourage everyone to bring the loving results of their self-care habits into their work-life and play-life routines, but reserve specific impressions for their love-life. An awakened self-concept can quite easily maintain harmony between all three aspects of life, as if a series of acts and scenes on a lifelong film are filled with real actors seeking genuine results.

Putting Self-Love Into Practice

How do we love ourselves? Sure, cheeky bubble-baths, social media positivity quotes, and muscle-bound mirror selfies show distinguished results concerning self-care habits. Considering that, when all the boxes are ticked: car, house, career, credit, security, and vacations, it's still possible to omit the commitment to loving ourselves. Letting ourselves experience joy, pleasure and happiness means we are finding ourselves piloting our intuition masterfully. Chemically, this means we are not addicted to dopamine rewards, but when we earn them, we celebrate them. Cursing under our breath, feigning affection, and ignoring negative self-talk can cast a dark shadow on an otherwise successful self-concept. Such symptoms are commonly associated with a never-live-up-to-my-expectations parental upbringing where shame and guilt hang heavily on the individual. The mission of many of us who aspire to act on these diagnoses is difficult when no clear circumstance exists to impress upon ourselves an inspiring, new way to live and love. The best that can be done sometimes is for us to act as a compass, directing the intuition into the pilot seat where although survival is the baseline of expectations, we always have hope—hope with habits of love.

Hope for ourselves is absolutely found next by setting goals. In fact, setting goals with someone important to us is indeed a good idea, but shouldn't over prioritize personal goals set for ourselves. Neither should we set goals simply for something to do. We are too spirited to be contained in someone else's goals or defined by a lack of enthusiasm on account of being cast in someone else's shadow. Fear of our true purpose amidst the bullying jealousy of lack luster ambition shouldn't be ignored. I know some clients when adopting new self-care habits were assaulted, traumatized, and set homeless when another was triggered and couldn't accept this newfound, empowered individual. So, busting down walls of insecurity should be done carefully and with subtle nonchalance. Be wise to incorporate friends and family with whom we recognize as welcoming self-love decisions. Be not afraid of discovering that when someone isn't ready to make a similar change as us, that they may react in complete denial. We should remember thus to act as the compass of survival and offer impressions that enable both neighbors and strangers to acknowledge up from down. My virgin sons taught me this in their youth. I was a rugby player and liked to offer my passion to my sons while they were young. My oldest twin, by a few minutes, instead took it upon himself to choose his own passion, that of baseball. His mission to make the triple A baseball team came through. I am thankful I found the ear to hear of his decision, and quickly supported him as he clearly loved pitching, batting, and winning as a team. I experienced with him how parents should welcome the origination of grand experiences that teach independence through responsible choices.

The foundation of the innocence of self-love is admired once we surmount the obstacles of survival and begin to thrive in our daily life. Jealousy, as a habit, debases our innocence and thwarts our goals, eroding our will to feel authentic and complete. Some of us may be searching for ways to thrive, and find ourselves scrolling social media, unable to formulate a will to take action from our desire. S.M.A.R.T. goals invite reality into the picture and take a broad desire only to transform it into practical actions. Someone with a self-concept who is determined to please others before themselves, is no doubt ridden with guilt for reasons unexplained. Familiar with someone setting their goals for them, they continue to do the same to others. It's an interesting economy to be sure, but also foolish since never was there an authentic invitation to be loved, only a desire to be given credit. Therefore, the judgment of results in the cycle of behavior should include self-love as a measurement of advantage over circumstances, not an advantage over others.

Loyalty to our self-care routine gives us character attributes that can be fortified despite periodic guilt trips and walks of shame. If ever asked to prove our love or loyalty to someone by sacrificing the love and loyalty we owe ourselves, remark how subtle the difference is. As both the foundation rock and corner stone are one and the same, we can find ourselves capable of being parents, fostering loving homes, and enjoying invitations for everlasting, loving romances, with complete security and protection.

CHECK

- I should identify what self-care means to me. I like to remember that my self-care ritual does not need to look like anyone else's. It just has to be one that brings me closer to achieving my goals.
- I should identify three self-care routines—one for each category of work, play and love—that I will perform every day regardless of the nature of my schedules—full or empty. I make sure these routines follow the template on building habits of love and incorporate S.M.A.R.T. goal guidelines so that I can effectively track myself over time.

6

LOVE MOVEMENT

Love is not what you say, love is what you do.

UNKNOWN

We all arrive on this earth as babies—oh, we were once so cute, young and fresh, born innocent with eyes opening for the first time, ready to grow and experience our first few breaths. Survival is taken for granted as a skill commonly misinterpreted for privilege, that many of us owe to our parents. My parents taught me the basics, and I learned the rest. Fortunate are those of us who enjoyed the peek-a-boos and birthdays, yet some of us may have missed those in favor of chores and the influence of things like cigarettes. Regardless of our past childhood, we are here now, reading this book and I am inviting us to look further inside ourselves, starting with the love of movement. So, let's admit to ourselves now that it's good to move a little bit.

The first part of adopting a love of movement is to remember how self-love is not about denying others from connecting with us. Hardly so. Self-love is about appreciating our self-worth. This is the measurement we have of ourselves, which we keep of ourselves, and we use in determining the importance of each moment, as it passes. Deciding to heal from past traumas, improves our self-worth. Remarking on the loving care our parents gave us, also improves our self-worth. Although the days pass by at the same rate for all of us, when we decide to experience each moment for everything it's worth, we are choosing to measure our life with great importance and great self-worth. So how do we use our knowledge of ourselves, with all of our cues and triggers, to create a cycle of behavior that lets us experience each moment in the best way possible? Do we need another love experiment? This sounds like a mystery. Well, a mystery it is indeed, one that we can unfold with deliberate efforts. This mystery is found when we remember to love ourselves first, with a love movement.

Although few of us find compensation as acrobats, high performing athletes, or supermodels, our physical bodies are still quite important to us. The regular use of our hands in coordination with our minds, our jaw and voice box in our speech, and our sense of smell which is altogether completely fascinating—are all parts of us we frequently take for granted. Yet still, when victimized by error and a cut thumb, a hoarse throat, or a nose numbing flu, we may deny how much we value our regular functions. This is too bad because we can formulate the frame of mind to be grateful, to practice gratitude. Gratitude formulates preventative habits, which help to maintain and enjoy the graces we are naturally born with. Since there is no warranty on body parts, and getting a new one is terribly impossible, we should examine the way we love our bodies using self-care habits. This part is not about our weight on the scale, nor our dream bikini body, or svelte abdominal line. We are evaluating the whole love for the body, from nose to toes.

Although negative thinking patterns affect us all, our self-worth is what we use to separate from those ill-conceived notions of anger, spite, and resentment. Did we once stub our toes? Maybe we found ourselves cursing under our breath with that sharp pain? "Who put that there?" we exclaim, or even worse. Forgiving ourselves of any foul language is not easy when pain is the dominant motivation of thought. Maybe foul language and foul thoughts have become normal to us. Who is in control of our words when we forget ourselves under moments of duress? Is it not us? In the scene of the psyche, deciding to act within the desires of others, that is, to cooperate and engage in life, in such a way so as not to undermine the boundaries of our own self-worth, will allow us to find advantage over temporary pain. I mean to say, the pain of humility. Yes, I have stubbed my toe, and I tried to blame the furniture and whoever put it there. Woefully wrong was I, and I dare say, I've learned it doesn't help me to waste my energy on negative emotions and thoughts. Instead, when we prepare ourselves with feelings of inspiration and thoughts of splendor, even for mundane things like putting the chair under the table, we realize we stumble over ourselves less and less. And, we certainly find how to value our self-worth, more and more. Less becomes more in the drama of the love movement. Any experience of ecstasy is first preceded by accepting humility.

This leads us to our face, which is generally the most vulnerable part of our body, and which we use quite extensively to communicate. From our face we communicate the majority of our states of mind—how we feel and react to ongoing events shows up through our facial expressions, something we actually rarely get to witness unless we pursue careers in film or modeling. Facial recognition is so important, we have a portion of our brain solely devoted to this task—the fusiform gyrus in the temporal lobe. Caring for our faces with scrubbing, exfoliating, and moisturizing is one thing indeed. But our faces also exude an aura that reveals our internal state. If we feel overly self-conscious, abusers may read our face as a victim to be had. In a job interview, it is not only the answers the interviewers are judging, but also the sincerity of a person, measured through their new, fresh face to the company. In relationships, especially intimate ones, the face is where much oily fluids are transmitted between lovers. When we hold stress, grief, anger & regret in our hearts, we will be preoccupied with these base level emotions and not only communicate them through our faces but leave lasting impressions on those around us. Because we live in a social context, it reasons to say that checking in the mirror and learning to love our face is an important key to acknowledging our impact on those around us. Because this reality influences all of us, it stands to say that our ability to react and reason with others relies on our ability to read the emotional expressions of those around us. To improve how we read faces, we need to logically understand these emotions within ourselves first. Only then can we empathize enough to build bridges of forgiveness, understanding and love with anyone.

Some people say that dog owners eventually share the same facial features as the dogs they own. Go figure. Emotional recognition is second to facial recognition in evaluating social reasoning. Besides our face then, our bodies communicate emotions through movement, speech and touch. If we observe the fluidity of our movements, we might discern our mood and state of mind. When triggered by someone cutting us off in traffic, our face might grimace, a foul word might pop out, and a first or jaw might clench. It's ok to observe these common reactions, but it's possible to observe our body react in a different way. For instance, with enough practice of smiling in the mirror, we might be predisposed to driving a little slower and letting people in, but, when tempted to react so enraged by the risk posed of an accident, we can instead channel that potent creative instinct of the brain stem to quickly exhale and step on the brake while studying the periphery for opportunity of escape. What this means is, if the point of exercise is to feel good about having a fit, able body, then that is only the first part.

We should be careful not to let ourselves fall into a drama that justifies itself to avoid setting and achieving goals, especially love goals. The practical nature of engaging with others, while maintaining principles of self-love requires that we remember ourselves from moment to moment. By accumulating sufficient efforts to engage in self-love habits, getting lost in conversation about nothing at all with someone new can still inspire us to laugh and form relationships we value. Deciding to appreciate ourselves, means our self-worth will grow exponentially the more we value it. Scenes of hate, indecision, and alpha-dominance will no longer draw us in, and instead our new scene of temperance and joy will let us become observers. The audience of the egotistical is there not to avoid the spotlight of leadership and accountability, but more so, to really recognize it within. Eventually, the opportunity to charge our energy levels up with self-love as our fuel, will become automatic—through habits of love.

The mystery of our mechanical nature is that self-love is determined by the association we make to everyday internal events. When internal circumstances are favorable, (we are happy) the ability to better enjoy external events is also favorable. In other words, our internal scene determines our ability to comprehend life as it happens around us. Self-love allows us to leverage the creative force within us to manufacture opportunity with desire. However, we get caught when we ignore the destructive opposite of the creative force, which is justifiably useful in finding opportunities. The balance of the two, creative and destructive, when we speak our will, and hear that of others, brings us into balance, into equilibrium.

This means that we have found how self-love as a concept requires us to understand the impermanence of ourselves on the earth—our mortality. Balancing thoughts of creation and destruction requires us to discern the difference between inspiration and letting go of the pain. Such decisiveness lets us find patterns of behavior we have, routines of emotional justification we use, and realities of grief we can't yet overcome as excuses to replace self-love. How sensible it would be to let go of pain, and what amazing results we will find! When we start accessing creative intelligence through intuitive inspirations, we manifest psychological states which match external environments, letting us handle life with grace and goodwill.

The second part of adopting a love of movement is to develop love habits of our body. As we know, the instinct to defend ourselves from danger, like a car accident, relies on how prepared we are to read a situation for favorable circumstances or outcomes. So, no matter how strong anyone gets, or how finely tuned in instinctive cognitions anyone trains, the love habit involved with training is what is reinforced. It's common to associate testosterone as the only measure of love in the intentions behind the results of a muscular athlete seeking to mate. Of course, this is organized by the agreement of an eligible mate to bond with. What is missed is the dance between Oxytocin and Testosterone in balancing the required empathy in caregiving for children, with the deliberate desire to mate. Many studies show that affection and attraction in the love habits of the body are regulated by hormones. These hormones are further understood, comprehended and controlled when we engage in regular exercise that challenges our state of mind around loving topics like caring for children and mating.

Higher Oxytocin contributes to being able to empathize with the problems of others. Oxytocin is fostered by and regulated with caring conversations with others, the practice of yoga, listening to delightful music, getting or giving a massage, spending time with others, aromatherapy and meditation. This is not an exhaustive list to say the least, but it should impact the idea within us to remember to have flexibility in being receptive to others' needs as well as to ours. This brings us to Testosterone, a mighty hormone important to both sexes.

Testosterone is important to regulate the sex drive, or libido, of men and also women to some degree. It's common between both sexes that by lifting weights, engaging in cardiovascular activities, eating high protein and high fat diets, along with low cortisol or low stress levels will lead to consistently high testosterone within the bloodstream. Only in women does testosterone combine with estrogen. But, again, it's common that without exercise, the right diet, and sufficient sleep, testosterone levels will be low, and the sex drive of individuals will decrease, as well as the satisfaction of the sexual act, as it may become mechanical.

The act of the love movement requires many scenes to come together to eventually form a film. This film is viewed 100% internally and our intuition is its only witness until we die. Start now by identifying moments in your life when you did feel love—love for yourself, love for family, love for friends, love for lovers, etc. Remember that your film has not ended, and that even if we are left with only memories, we should digest those memories, and remember ourselves as having earned them. With the film still playing on the screen of our mind, we realize quickly how valuable we are to our loved ones, and to ourselves—only then we can realize what opportunity awaits us in the near future. Journal it, speak it, love it. We should find ourselves awakened tomorrow morning, with goals we want to achieve, as a person we want to be.

FINDING THE DISCIPLINE

Research suggests that two things determine whether we would commit to our love movement routines—a perception of competence and control (Teixeira et al, 2012). When we feel we are competent, and when we believe we control our own exercise method, schedule, and intensity, our habits of the body tend to be much more consistent. If we are coming from an athletic background, we should continue to temper our routines with habits of love added in. If we are just getting started, we need to bring our love habits to whatever love movement we choose and set foundations of sincere practice with goals.

Motivation and discipline are different perspectives but distinct stages of loving moving. While social media posts and encouraging words from friends or spouses will motivate anyone to take on goals of better exercise routines, the ultimate motivator is ourselves. The difference, as you, no doubt, realize, is that inner motivation becomes a discipline when it's met with action in the real world. Every one of us, as individuals, must forge new patterns of behavior that become disciplines unique to our love goals.

Yes, partnering with people is vital to enjoying life in general, especially the love movement of exercise since the discipline doesn't feel so regimented when we forget the reason why we came and just learn to enjoy people's company. Of course, the motivation should be consistent with the discipline so as to know how to read the social environment. We should take cues from others, set our desires, communicate our goals, and build patterns we are going to be proud of. It will show in our faces if we honestly want to break new barriers and enter new social scenes.

All of our habits of the body can be observed by remarking on its novel capabilities. I know in my youth I had the metabolism of what seemed like a young tiger, but as I've observed my relationship with age, I've had to refine my feelings of invincibility to still abide in the glory of this flesh and bones container. We should allow ourselves to embark on the journey of exercise and its love movement because biologically the results are definitely beneficial. Even one day per week for one hour at a time, when given 12 weeks to adjust to our routine will offer harmonious benefits in our hormones, delivering insight into an inner journey for companionship, resulting in the opportunity to face social interactions where we can observe further our desire to achieve fulfillment. It will show up in our faces. Naturally, exercise, when formulated with the intuitive frame of mind to descend into the cycle of behavior, will turn into a constant affair with other aspects of our life, like nutrition, thought patterns, and emotional associations—associations of the soul.

In our beautiful body, we are enriched with muscles and joints, organs and hormones, blood and water, air and excrement. Obviously, handling our body requires us to respect it, just as we respect the red and green lights of traffic signals on the street. When we are in tune with our daily self-care practices of our love movement, love habits will result in as much as we are prepared to do them. Since our muscles and joints act only in a flexion or relaxation, we need to purposefully find a way to awaken the potential of muscular and joint extension through stretching—cognitive relaxation. Just as our daily self-care routines are sometimes found to be needing improvement, so is our love movement. More and more strength only contributes to reinforce the directive of setting goals and achieving them. While this is the aim of S.M.A.R.T. goals to build strength and resolve, we should also temper our ambitions with stretching as our intention is to enjoy the practice of achieving them.

Stretching allows our muscles and joints to heal and recuperate after use, making them more useful later on in their performance. When depleted, muscles and joints need rest. They also need blood, and time to generate cells with that blood. Further, they need to remove wastes from their regeneration, to allow new cells the space they need to form. Stretching also opens up cells for the flow of blood, controlled by the parasympathetic nervous system. Sometimes, stretching then releases endorphins as a part of the body's natural reward system. These rewards of stretching accentuate and reinforce positive emotions. This whole stretching process is a receptive practice of the feminine perspectives of habits of love. While strength and conditioning are masculine derivatives, stretching is the feminine counterpart. We should accept both in our resilience and resolve in our love movement principles. Now, as we stretch our minds and learn to become more receptive to any new feelings we have about movement and exercise, here are pertinent checks to cash related to loving our body.

CHECK

- I should identify the reasons I have for the exercises I do already. Some of these habits are already ingrained into my daily affairs, and I will probably find hard to give up as they form the foundations of my hormonal cycles.
- I should list three rewards from exercise that I'd like to experience, and I won't hold back. I need to be clear with myself, so I use S.M.A.R.T. goals as a tool since they allow me to break down how I should achieve my desired rewards. For instance, it's helpful not to ignore that if I want to do that motorcycle tour with my spouse for two weeks, I will have to be physically fit to endure the road tests. The reward is therefore broken into three parts: confidence in making the trip, joy in the romance of it happening, and gratitude for being prepared. Confidence, joy, gratitude—maybe this will turn out to be a yearly habit that I love doing with my spouse? It's surprising how I can actually achieve the results I want when I have the leverage of love to intelligently do so.
- I should find out within my exercise goals, how love plays a part—no, not lust, love. With a foundation of love in my heart, despite any soreness, I can conquer pain with resilience. This doesn't require too much investment on the front end, an hour a week to start is pretty good, but on

the back end, this investment of time can be undermined. As cortisol is the stress hormone, when I stay up late, overcommit to others, I lose sleep, have irregular routines, and find an overall lack of sincerity in the exercise, lowering my testosterone and oxytocin levels. Then I might drop into my bad habits, returning to unconscious descending spirals of unfortunate circumstances without any advantage to gain from front end investments.

- To balance this back end heavy situation, I need to prepare my nutrition to balance my devotion to myself. This lets me handle the mental struggle that comes with making and achieving goals, so that I may integrate my spirit through soulful objectivity. Then I weigh circumstances to avoid overreacting. Stretching my body is a habit of love movement I see all over the world—from cats and dogs, to us as humans. It represents my being open to balanced nutrition, positive thoughts, and soulful life concepts. So, I should choose three stretches to enjoy, and to see if I can tell what anxieties or fears I can unlock within into those tight muscles and joints as I do them.

7

LOVE EATING WELL

"When you love what you have, you have everything you need."

UNKNOWN

Knowing that we all have wishes to feel good in our well-exercised bodies, establishing the perfect sense of nutrition to meet that wish is not always easy—it does take effort. What it starts with is to love eating. Even closer to the mark is to love feeding ourselves. The difference? Read on. From the associated virtue that all mothers have in their breast milk, we have learned that by providing tenderness to ourselves, we can feel nourished without too much complication. Much is spoken about new diets compared to the Standard American Diet (SAD) and my opinion is very up to date—we should take the time to know ourselves and choose wisely.

Not everything comes from the divine source of the mother's bosom, sadly. Holistically, choosing foods that align with our values is essential to loving ourselves. The vegetarian who doesn't eat meat, shouldn't resent the cattle rancher. The Vegan who avoids eggs, shouldn't get frustrated by the tax refunds issued to the chicken farms. Essentially knowing what we like and why is a large part of understanding our consumption habits.

When someone bites into their favorite meal, what are they eating, really? A murderous dictator with ruthless abandon experiences hunger just as anyone would. What brought him or her to be convinced of such a way of life, comes down from which impressions he or she chose to eat from. We generally feed off our environment—the delight it provides is conditional to its makeup. Living in a cave with no light, or in a lovely cabin within a valley of sunshine are two distinct impressions. How we survive and thrive in each depends on our frame of mind to transform the impression to benefit our psychological state.

Since our lives are dynamic and filled with people and places, things and sounds, words and faces, we have much to choose from about what and who impressed us most favorably. It's from these favorable impressions that we should eat, shouldn't we? Why eat from impressions of anger or over intellectualization? We should employ intuition to practice intuitive eating. My example is illustrious and farfetched, yet these stark contrasts help us to categorize our foods according to the mystery within them. What this cake means to you, is different from what it means to anyone else depending on where someone else is on the self-care journey in habits of love. A better and more realistic example is found in common, everyday practice: a cute co-worker is making passes at lunch looking for a date, he flirts with her, while she remembers her boyfriend packed her a lunch, still hidden under the table. Although it's tempting to eat from temporary flattery and arousal, as sometimes we should, the best impressions to love eating well should be judged according to our faith in our values. The values are established as we effectively set and work to achieve our S.M.A.R.T. love goals.

As it is quoted,

"When you love what you have, you have everything you need."

Knowing ourselves is the key to handling the hunger for life. The desire to love what we don't have yet is ok, as goals are necessary to give direction for what we want, but the habit of always loving what we have already alleviates the stress of striving for something else. Loving what we have can also surprise us in three ways. First by recognizing the marvelous human body—how it exists in the world is truly cosmic. Second, by recognizing we have parts of our lives we can't change (ie. our family) we can make choices with love as our guide towards things we can (ie. to start our own family). Third, what we truly 'eat' are impressions—like a constant river flowing through our five senses, we choose which impressions to act upon. We have only to transform the impressions we receive to truly realize how we are already getting what we need.

TRANSFORMATION OF IMPRESSIONS

All the impressions we experience are filtered through our five senses: sight, touch, hearing, smell, and taste. It's through these input channels that we can leverage love to improve our ability to transform impressions. For example, what we once found uncomfortable and even unconscionable can become, with enough love, normal and enjoyable. If we transform impressions regularly, we can study innocent feelings of queasiness, butterflies in the stomach, and 24-hour flus for what they are—moments of indecision based on new experience or important choices to be made.

As adults, as we adopt and perform self-care habits, our ability to filter impressions and lovingly transform them contributes to healthy gut microbiomes where food is digested. This is the same place where serotonin is produced, which influences our brains, and elegantly regulates our moods and behaviors.

Thankfully, the serotonin of women increases as romantic relationships ensue, concluding that the endearment between couples should reflect a woman's ability to handle her desires to mate with a consistent mood. Men, on the other hand, experience a drop in serotonin, indicating a vulnerability to control their moods. However, this is generally balanced by the increase of testosterone, which is like the workhorse hormone of the desire to breed with a mate.

To love eating well is a paradigm that is essential for couples to build on their strengths and to handle their weaknesses. This is especially true for single people who are recovering from previous traumas, setting new love goals. As dips and dives in moods occur, we realize that we are alone to transform impressions and should double up our self-care regimen. When couples combine self-care efforts with empathy for each other, finding foods to love eating well promotes habits of love to grow twice or three times as fast.

CHECK

- I start by making a list of what's in my fridge and cupboards, and describe why I like it, even love it. If the words cheap, convenient, and simple are used often, these are actually the words I am using to describe my life. I take no judgment; I just observe what I say. Finding a way to describe the ingredients in my meals with clarity, adoration, and gratefulness will inherently nourish myself in a completely different way.
- I shop or harvest my foods with a new list of words to describe my love of eating well. With a clarity and passion defined in my S.M.A.R.T. love goals, I find inspiration in combining eating habits with habits of love.
- I find a plant or herb that I can grow at home. If it's just the air we share, so be it, but if I can enjoy a sweet pepper or apple, I have transformed the impression of the food without marketing campaigns doing it for me.

8

LOVE THE SPIRIT

At the end of life, what really matters is not what we bought, but what we built; not what we got, but what we shared; not our competence, but our character; and not our success, but our significance.

UNKNOWN

What does a doctorate or licensure achieve in guaranteeing the efficacy or certainty of our habits of love? Neither having a Ph.D. nor not having one employs the love-result we are objectively targeting, nor do they prove anything about one's ability to experience love. Professional designations merely institute the lifelong scene, whereby self-respect is garnered through our comprehension of reality in society. Reality is just things as they are today for all of us.

Our spirit, therefore, recognizes accolades cognizant of our need to behave within society, but judges only through merits of the heart which are realized intuitively. Our spirit is the part of our psyche that realizes we can only live one life at a time. Not two or three lives, just one. The jealous want the lives of the other, unable to value the life they have. Our ability to value the love we can foster within ourselves allows us to avoid sabotaging opportunity. It's ok to wine and dine with temptation, but opportunity is no doubt what our spirit is here to help us with.

Only when we have fallen to temptation enough times and bottomed out completely, will we learn to remember to love the spirit sufficiently. As having learned our lessons from the point before we loved our spiritual self, to the moment after when we did, we will find our spirit as the wind beneath our wings. Always obeying the airflow of opportunity, never submitting to the sands of trying to manipulate others, we can enjoy the spiritual pursuit of independent decisions. Harking to the advantage of the spiritual self over the pragmatic personality, it's found that habits of love are all the difference.

Knowing that our personality is composed of a multitude of characteristics is wonderful—intelligence, imagination, wittiness, curiosity, humor, empathy, compassion, and so on. Perhaps we have categorized ourselves into INFJ or something else and we feel satisfied with these categorizations since we have already decided that we are shy, sarcastic, or a visual learner. That's fine, but maybe we haven't and I'm not saying we have to. What the personality and the rational mind are limited to are irrational ideas which can only be handled by the spirit. Conquering love of the spirit is akin to earning independence from our parents, and the associated pre-dispositions of our youth, while also handling the throes of survival as we enjoy life to its maximum before we eventually reach our death bed. Knowing what the responsibilities of life are is indeed important to guaranteeing we live in good spirits with peace of mind, and without fear of morbidity. Some say that when we satisfy our responsibilities in life we achieve a child-like state of awareness—a sort of return to innocence. Love and the lust of sex are two more components we should handle with this innocent moment of spiritual awareness. The reality is our love of spirit offers our personality limitless options for refinement through love and sex as we habitually feed it with its source of nourishment—faith.

Sufficient rebelliousness, and ultimate devotion are innate qualities that surface and grow, like roots in healthy soil with sun and libations of rain, despite temptation. That is, it's possible to actually welcome opportunity from temptation. It is aghasting, oftentimes, how skillful the heart is to renounce bad habits, when the substantial flavor of our love of spirit is tasted instead. Our cycle of behavior, when governed by the love of spirit, is nourished by the transformation of impressions; that is, when a candid thought from a perceived failure is quickly re-interpreted, we have opportunity in disguise. Fair weathered friends, no doubt, could be still seeking the love for the spiritual self. Any measurement of the spirit, for that matter, is actually immeasurable. Forgiveness, therefore, of the fair weathered friend, is a mighty tool in the realm of transformation. With the love spirit, life is small compared to the enormity of time and space. But, with the spirit we should accomplish great things anyways, or else get lost in analyzing how the grass is greener on the other side.

The love of spirit, therefore, serves two modalities. Its ultimate feature is a divine sense of purpose, which includes emotional fulfillment and right judgment. But interestingly, it inspires good will, which forces newer and more innovative ways for self-expression. Clearly, inspiring spiritual love endows others to do the same, but it is incomplete until they themselves recognize their independence wholeheartedly.

Such is the reward of opportunity from temptation; it is always gratifying as it only besets the mystery of the moment.

The secret of learning our own sexual mystery, reminds us how sometimes, when sparks jump from flint and a keen eye is met with equal wonder we have an authentic connection. Other times, authenticity is a target only for the mythical Achilles to find. Habits of love requires practice to find the marksman of our individually destined journey to love the spirit. Part IV of this book introduces the measurements of practice, but before that we still have facets of ourselves to investigate and survey. Let's relax, be grateful, and begin.

CHECK

- I create a list of love goals that have spiritual significance to me—love goals I place my faith in. I usually transform them into S.M.A.R.T. goals to go and achieve, but which I can adopt every day, with an openness about it so that I can explain it to others.
- These love goals should include things like: how do I feel about fasting? Do I believe in sex before marriage? Do I want to experience other countries and other cultures? What do I expect out of marriage? Having children? Visiting grave sites? Attending church? Giving spiritual lessons? As I define these spiritual love goals, I will value the decisions I make today as I begin realizing them.

9

LOVE REST

"I love you not because of who you are, but because of who I am when I am with you."

ROY CROFT

We have found the ability to discern the balance between our creative and destructive halves. While exercising to stretch our minds and love our bodies, we've seen how to nourish ourselves according to our sexes, all while activating our digestive comprehension to leverage love in moment-to-moment impressions—impressions we give and impressions we receive. This intuitive combination of loving attitudes reassures us that we can fulfill our spirit with the self-love principle.

What desires we may have had which were keeping us triggered into old habits, have now been tempered by a separation from scenes we were previously stuck within. By refining our desires, we remove any animal instinct to rip, tear or claw, and replace it with the human condition to love, love, and love. This is organized and cultivated into society not only because of morality, but for our true potential to be unleashed. Animal desires undermine our cycle of behavior causing us to intellectualize, over think, and waste time.

Instead, we should use intuitive qualities to inspire passion now, now, now, to choose an all-in-one lifetime experience.

This way, we are much more inclined to accept forgiveness as the root for achieving advantage over judgment in resolutions of love. This means that when judging others for not loving us back, we must clearly require ourselves to stop interpreting their existence that way. However, it is not ignorant to refrain from committing to loving someone without them accepting our love in the same way we value ourselves.

For example, we may be jealous of the criminal who uses love and receives affection under the umbrella of organized cycles of behavior. But this is the same tool the Police use in their organized processes. Thus, we can rest easily knowing that corruption need not be entertained as the guide of the spirit, despite the persuasion of the drama it inspires. In fact, any matters of consistent efforts and practical means in self-love habits will permit our waters of creation to quench our thirst with the initiative of just-thought and just-emotion.

Regarding the saving of energy and the value of our time, we just love rest and relaxation. When we choose our battles for the maintenance of our habits of love we give ourselves the chance of faithfully pursuing satisfaction. This personal satisfaction can also be admired in others as we reach and achieve some goals, without worrying about the ones we didn't achieve. This common ground between opposing forces of creation and destruction leverages love to be the measurement of success and best results—which interestingly lets criminals fall prey to the same law of love. We all judge so faithfully together to love rest and relaxation that despite who we have been told to be, it is what we actually do that matters.

Sometimes the best we can do is nothing at all, or more aptly, if we have nothing good to say, say nothing at all. Loving rest is serendipity and serenity, where coincidence always follows. When we find time to enjoy a quiet mind we attract harmony, especially in quiet moments of intimacy. After analyzing the temperament of my mind, I've learned that if I do not rest and relax, my thoughts will get the best of me, and I'll become grumpy with those around me who I love oh so dearly. Why would anyone let this happen? The stress of expectation and responsibility can be a heavy burden to keep organized when love feels chaotic and complicated. Learning to simplify is therefore the exercise of this chapter on loving to rest. How rest and relaxation are best found to compliment love is entirely when the heart has harnessed and tempered the mind. The contemplative heart needs to be exercised and not forgotten nor ignored.

When complete adoption of a love to rest occurs, the cue and trigger towards bad habits take less and less hold on our psyche, permitting greater faith in love as a discipline overall. Although sex may be the motivation, unless love is its discipline, sex too can lead to a disorganization of partnerships between couples, exactly when consent isn't present. So, love rest because it doesn't matter how much self-love we promise ourselves—a sore-back, or painful hip upsets us. We should therefore always find practical actions to rest with self-love acknowledgments in-line with our desired results.

CHECK

These three rest exercises can be done once a week for an hour, or daily for ten minutes all together before leaving the house.

- I use this quote By Roy Croft as a mantra in my mind "I love you not because of who you are, but because of who I am when I am with you." (Quote Catalog, n.d.) and when my mind is settled, I breathe calmly for two minutes, and proceed to the next exercise. Remember that the benefits of our love to rest and relax start with sleep: Eight hours per night allows my body to heal itself, allows me to enjoy my dreams, builds confidence in my sense of self, helps me to avoid being triggered by bullies, traffic, and illness, and permits me to originate new thinking patterns and new emotions.

- I sit and relax in a chair, close my eyes and envision hearing myself talk using words of self-love. Literally I should talk to myself in my mind with affirming words of affection and admiration for the qualities I should congratulate myself with. Words I use on myself are the same I end up using on others too.

- I envision further words I'd use with others, modeled as desired words I'd say to myself in a complete conversation. Known as "paving" this sets the movement of my 'plane' of thought for the day or week, to move about gracefully with others as I pilot my life between 'flights.' When faced with circumstances I am surprised of, this "paving" prepares not just my mind, but actually my emotions mostly. I become receptive and react with genuine care, exhibiting authentic empathy, maintaining an amazing integrity behind my intentions and complete confidence that my words will be there for me when the scene arrives.

10

LOVE GRATITUDE

Love doesn't make the world go 'round, love is what makes the ride worthwhile.

FRANKLIN P. JONES

Anyone who sets goals is beginning to crystallize into reality what they are truly aiming to achieve. The conscious choice of writing and formulating ideas into projections for the future delivers intention for the ultimate aim of fulfillment. Intentions themselves are measured in tandem with results because by maintaining intentions we can evaluate the journey for its level of experience. When we remember a dream, we are developing a restful quality of emotional temperance that is a quiet remembering of our self-concept, an amazing result from habits of love through a love of rest.

The innocence of newborn children is mesmerizing, but there should also be an appreciation for the wisdom of our elders. Between the ages of 20 to 80 and beyond, there aren't many changes happening to the outer shell of our bodies, except for gray hairs and a few wrinkles. Our understanding of the grandiosity of life should therefore be appreciated early and valued through the many years we will share together. For this reason, love can be found at any moment, regardless of age. Choosing to build on that love requires us to be grateful we've found it.

But what can be said about goals we set to challenge ourselves, individually or as couples? What about fears we uncover as we face the uncertain future with our desire for certainty? Trying to relax and adopt another self-love habit requires our bills to be paid, the children's mouths to be fed, and the car to start in the morning. If this is so, then it must be said that only in self-defense would we be interested in rejecting the foul intentions of anyone. When clear indications of threats and bullying behaviors are signaling or indicating aggression to our person, we should guard our intentions to not find our desires twisted and manipulated. A mounting terror of change occurs when someone identifies with what is going on and feels singled out. With an example of an aggressor who wishes to bust some knuckles, it is terribly difficult to see things as they are before trying to persuade things to be the way we desire them to be without conflict. To disarm an opponent with a mounted defense we would need to see, hear and feel how they are frightfully weak and insecure in their self-love capabilities and do so with empathy.

Being grateful for what opportunities we have available to us permits us to avoid the traps set by the pain we feel, our memories left undigested, and any hurtful words still lingering in our minds. Patience is this lovely tool which we use to gauge our gratefulness. Patience lets us work at setting the scene for advantageous opportunities to achieve results like safety, integrity, respect, which allows our habits of love to foster. Ultimately, everyone is trying to gain advantage over circumstances, we are wired this way, but short-sightedness sometimes proves that unless we are grateful, we'll get stuck. I know that when I transform the impressions of an abuser, I realize how grateful I am to become more self-secure. I love gratitude as I form a boundary and recognize my independence because of it.

Giving ourselves the acknowledgment that what we are attracting is a reflection of our internal state reassures us that we should take ourselves seriously but gently as we avoid reproach for the world at large. Who we are is only as important to us as we make it out to be. There are two realizations from loving gratitude we can ultimately discover. First, someone has decided to love us, as they love themselves—a classic example of a loving relationship between two independent people. And secondly, we might realize how we are in a one-sided relationship where love hasn't yet been found by the other. K. Tonloe wisely said,

"Sometimes the right way to love, is to leave."

K. TOLNOE (ARTOFIT, N.D.)

Who we are depends not on how we might feel about ourselves when we're reading this, but more about who we are after. To love gratitude is to remember who we were before we discovered habits of love. This also matters just as much. Letting someone discover for themselves how they are going to be grateful for what they have is essential in knowing we truly have our independence. Right now, I imagine the very best for us, I really do, and I would love to see us at our very best. So, we should love ourselves, because if not this book is just a weight in our hands resting on our laps. I try to charge it with the very intention of inspiring everyone, of all stripes, in the relentless aim of realizing our potential to love and to be loved in return. So, let's do it, and not look back. Let's earn the rewards of tying these love-me-knots and be grateful as we humbly protect ourselves.

Be not small in dreams and reach high, well beyond expectations. To love gratitude is to also realize we have done enough for the day so that we can rest well, ready to pave the way for tomorrow. That way, as our dreams touch our heart, we will find our true potential is set free by those who would do us harm—physically, emotionally, or psychologically. As we cast them out or leave on our own independently, we love gratitude as we recognize the major internal change taking place. This means we should find passion in sexual affairs and be bridled by the genuine adventure of the intuition. But, because of gratefulness, we shouldn't be preoccupied with who gets the last laugh. There are just too many people to love, so instead, stay inspired and be genuine with every step as we pilot the next act in the film of our life, loving ourselves first. In this life-long film, therefore, we can truly experience a love for everyone.

CHECK

These two exercises are complimentary, but each has their own specific aim in so far as gratefulness. Try the first and go onto the second.

- If ever I feel physically dominated or threatened, I should visualize using words like "get out," "leave" and "stop" to feel empowered. As I remember myself and to avoid choking on the opportunity, I should say these few words in person or report to the authorities, of course, kindly and with loving urgency. Valuing my personal space allows me to experience gratefulness for what I have and to feel protected with just-action.

- One person cannot accomplish the love of two. It isn't selfish to admit where the boundaries of a relationship need to be drawn. I consider people I have loved very much and establish with them how I expect to be treated, naturally, based on how I love myself. This practice of maintaining a self-image isn't paradoxical, it's for clarity. After all, this may reveal how I can strengthen my resolve to be independent, carry out my commitments to myself, and start making my commitments to others. I know now, it's okay to share commitment with others in their journey to also becoming independent.

PART IV

LIVING HABITS OF LOVE

The measure of time spent loving ourselves or loving someone else becomes vain when we realize it should be a constant habit, formulated to engender happiness and goodwill for our entire life, until we take our last breath. The gratitude of each moment, inspired by this opportunity of constant love, enables an abundance of love to flow from within and without promoting health and individuality. Living with habits of love therefore permits us to do the impossible: love others before they know how, protect ourselves despite our shortcomings, and hold faithful to a spirit of forgiveness, so that our spiritual enlightenment may ultimately take root, benefiting our lives this very minute. I offer three practices to integrate into the film of our lives, which should offer a wholesome summary of all that we have learned in this book so far—chapter over chapter, check over check, exercise over exercise.

11

PRACTICE BEING AN EMPTY CUP

There is only one happiness in this life, to love and be loved.

GEORGE SAND

In our early childhood, we may remember the innocence of when we didn't know about a sore-back, taxes, or thievery. Life was resplendent then, and, maybe even more so now that we are using habits of love to heal from any childhood traumas. Using memories of embracing our parents, opening Christmas presents, and enjoying family meals, helps us to celebrate our innocence. This innocence is our innate curiosity, totally free from judgment. This innocence is also emblematic of an empty cup—always ready to be filled with knowledge, brimming with excitement. We may have spilled this cup once or twice, making a few mistakes and accidents along the way, but it's both expected and easily forgiven of children.

Because of these few spills, we, as children, had a heavy dependence on our parents. Never did we conceive that we were taking anything for granted. Naturally, this child-like point-of-view changes as the seasons change and we grow up, but the traditions of holidays and their messages to children don't. Tradition reserves forgiveness for the innocent in the inevitable mistakes we are going to make, through lessons. Lessons actually taught by Santa, the Easter bunny, St.

Valentine, that imply forgiveness. Get on the good list, enjoy cute and cuddly feelings, and faithfully love someone. This goes on as our traditions reveal results when we commemorate the resilience of fostering a spirit of coursing on through, learning on the go, from our mistakes. To name a few, we have Thanksgiving, for its harvesting of not just food, but goodwill; Independence Day, for its realizations of freedom, but also individuality; and Veterans Day, when the brave are remembered, and celebrations of gallantry understood.

And so, we should fill up our cup as a daily self-care practice, but also remember to wake up with it empty, so as to be ready to fill it up again. When we think we have learned all of the traditions from our culture, let's look again, go a little deeper, and see how tradition reaches further back than technology. It has always been love, driving us forward, innovating our minds, both young or old, to be a little better, feel more genuine, and aim a little higher.

Such ideas of being an empty cup draw on the facets of the wisdom of love. Wisdom, generally associated with old age, comes with an abundance of patience, am I right? Sometimes, people of old age get to speak of how they conquered physical pain, reaped financial success, and outwitted the criminal. Children remind us of the wisdom of achieving those ends. If not for the stories and traditions of life as we have lived it, we might forget the novelty of experiencing life as it happens. Children are loving and often express love unconditionally, especially when we love them and treat them as we should. For this reason, I say it's ok to make mistakes, so long as we practice being an empty cup. The practice to adopt this habit of love into our daily life is to place an empty cup inside a box or cupboard, and to keep it safe whether it's locked away in secret or left on display. Write a note, place it inside the cup that reads, "I will always love you," and tap into the perspective of always doing so. In this way, the saying, "you can't pour from an empty cup" is used to differentiate between the clutter of a busy mind, and the authentic attitude of a full heart.

12

PRACTICE UNTIL PERFECT

Love doesn't need to be perfect, it just has to be true.

UNKNOWN

The oxymoron of this chapter is that the practice of trying to achieve perfection is possible, but the achievement of perfection itself is a letdown we must simply tolerate. I phrase this in such a way as to imply a complete annihilation of expectation that anyone besides ourselves will solve our problems of love but us. We can trust that we have as much time on this Earth as anyone else, and it's now our goal to simply love everyone unconditionally just as our father and mother loved us through our conception.

Loving our parents is a unique birthright, which I encourage everyone to understand. When we do—mere sounds, sights, movements, tastes of food, great company, and great ideas, result in the development of our intimate character. When these facets of our character shine brilliantly, we should take the opportunity of such perfection and realize the love we have for ourselves in order to share it with others. When we don't, our passions will peter out and we'll be stuck with regret. That is, unless we do the following: source inspiration over comfort, imagination over disinterest, and intuition over intellectualization. These three signs of fatigue, when remedied, balance our efforts through substantive actions—

actions to give and receive love. These remedies are true measurements we've found that result in changing bad habits from getting worse, to love habits getting better.

Being powerful is a practice of perfection, although only poignantly, since being shy shouldn't undermine anyone's ability to be present. By following the practices in this book, we learn to command this sense of presence. So go ahead, gather in book clubs, and discuss these topics of love together. Open up with each other knowing that the way forward is mysterious, yet it requires practical preparations. Be intuitive, not impulsive—exact temperance and define boundaries, yet explore desires and feed the imagination. When we learn to begin every day with the idea of fulfilling our goals, we perceive what's possible for us. As our intentions are measured and put into action, our bravery armors our resolve to follow through. We should awaken ourselves to great friendships, compassionate colleagues, and encouraging adults—directing traffic to the fluidity of romance and sexual exploration. Manifesting these valuable ideals won't be short lived, but it will be tested—illnesses, trouble, disaster, denial, grief, temptation—all amount to realities we need to face. These are times when the world values our decision to use love the most.

It's because we know mistakes happen, humiliations occur, and crime victimizes everyone, that we should prepare for it, witness it, and accept the challenge to prevent it. When we do all this with habits of love, we are committing to the integration of a core of beliefs that transcends racial boundaries, amplifies the voice of minority groups, and exercises healing strategies for the traumatized. Habits of love are truly very powerful, although they also require the perfect faith in the subtle strength of a butterfly's wings.

13

PRACTICE MINDFULNESS

Live the life you love, love the life you live.

BOB MARLEY

Living with a generous heart is the nature of the abundance of love. When realizing how to abide in such abundance we practice the exercise of mindfulness. We are often thwarted by attempts at adding variations in our routines, which prove a lack of consistency in our self-care habits. For example, an hour of self-care doesn't justify 30-minutes of negative self-talk, nor gossiping. Yet, it's ok to catch and observe our own ill-natured behaviors. They are merely reminders that less is more.

A simple routine that lasts only ten weeks proves so much compared to a complicated one—one that goes for gusto and falls short. A behavior cycle that descends to the root of issues, eventually funnels tenderness, like a truth serum, straight to the heart, and which we are all eventually bound to find and enjoy very very much.

Mindfulness is an appreciation for the reserve of attention we keep for the intuition to function properly. Inevitably, our capacity to comprehend the beautiful organization of nature, including all human nature, resides within our faith in love, using intuition.

Mindfulness exemplifies the higher intelligence of hunches, rationalizations of gut feelings, and dedicated progressions of skills towards mastery. With confidence and enough practice anyone who wishes to experience abundance, experiences the wealth of love.

At this point, love could be described as an island, where at first, we might feel limited by its incredible requirement to be both righteous and selfless amidst the bounds of the limited shoreline of our time on earth.

But finally, with the wisdom of practice, we realize that despite our hesitancy towards responsibility, the island of love ultimately provides entertainment for our soul to invoke chemistry and add romance giving unlimited potential to our life. Therefore, I say again to start using love in our cycle of behavior now. By unshackling our minds from the triggers of bad habits we regain the novelty of an empty cup and begin the routine of handling the added vitality that comes with habits of love.

Many delightful hormones result in wonderful thoughts and feelings, enlightening our minds to happiness, and growing our hearts hand over fist. The really difficult task is maintaining our integrity and honoring our words. It is tempting to try to do too much once we feel the surge of sexual energy coming from the understanding that anything is possible. We must continue to set boundaries as we set our goal-oriented love priorities.

There will be periods when it might be tough to avoid giving up. Signs of giving up are dropping the expectations of our

S.M.A.R.T. love goals, ignoring the crossing of our boundaries, and giving into the temptation of trying to do too much to please everybody. If we stick to our self-care preparations and trust that it is truly worth knowing ourselves, then as we observe our habits and learn to make goals based on what we want to achieve, we are making great strides.

When we have to say "no" because we haven't any more to give, we should let any feelings of guilt dissipate as we rest and relax remembering to be grateful. Saying "yes" to ourselves is then the decision to let our own love experiment take place, because that is the mindful understanding of the glory of love, where our faith shines brilliantly through the silent love exuded in our face.

CONCLUSION

HABITS OF LOVE CAN BE FOUND EVERYDAY

The greatest happiness of life is the conviction that we are loved; loved for ourselves, or rather, loved in spite of ourselves

VICTOR HUGO

Inevitably, many of our habits were derived from the education we received from our parents at a young age. Family, friends, peers, and colleagues who may have impressed upon us, have no doubt influenced our behaviors still. As an adult, most of our habits are found originally as a means of survival, but can lead further, to allow us to thrive to unlimited ends.

What we've discovered about ourselves is that by performing self-care checks within our daily routine of self-observation, we can pilot our life to find advantages over circumstances where we previously saw none. As we discipline ourselves to smartly define our desires, we can filter good from bad, deciding which habits we want to keep, leveraged with cues to act lovingly. Feeling prepared to balance love in all areas of our life, it's clear the abundance of love is ever present, and to access it we should descend into the deepest depths possible within ourselves.

Loving to eat and nourish ourselves, coupled with the joy of movement, expression, sights and sounds, is completely electrifying and rewarding. This appreciation reinforces self-love as a motto, whereby we are reminded to also rest, relax, and balance our initiative with receptivity. Practicing habits of love is therefore a complete affair of the heart, where our intuition gets all the glory as it partners with our intimate spirit. Both couples and single people experience love, and all of us should dedicate our lives to it, day-in and day-out.

ABOUT DAN HARTMAN

This simple book is written for everyone and will hopefully be translated into as many languages as possible. Take a moment now to feel happy about having read it and pass it on to everyone you know. The best way to start your movement into habits of love, is to write a 5-star review, or post a VLOG while tagging us with #habitsoflove so as tell us how you found love in your heart from reading it. I can be reached at:

Dan.hartman@intuitive-way.com

REFERENCES

A-Z Quotes. (n.d.-a). Albert Ellis quote. A-Z Quotes. Retrieved April 7, 2022, from https://www.azquotes.com/quote/88681

A-Z Quotes. (n.d.-b). Denis Waitley quote. A-Z Quotes. Retrieved April 7, 2022, from https://www.azquotes.com/quote/810141

A-Z Quotes. (n.d.-c). Randy Gage quote. A-Z Quotes. https://www.azquotes.com/quote/1139121

Artofit. (n.d.). We sometimes the right way to love is to leave K. Tolnoe. Artofit. Retrieved April 7, 2022, from https://www.artofit.org/image-gallery/620511654906904859/we-sometimes-the-right-way-to-love-is-to-leave-k-tolnoe-ifunny/

Berk, L. E. (2018). Development through the lifespan (7th ed.). Pearson.

Brainy Quote. (n.d.). Franklin P. Jones quotes. BrainyQuote. Retrieved April 8, 2022, from https://www.brainyquote.com/quotes/franklin_p_jones_142113#:~:text=Jones%20Quotes&text=Please%20enable%20Javascript-

Catron, M. L. (2015, January 9). To fall in love with anyone, do this (published 2015). The New York Times. https://www.nytimes.com/2015/01/11/style/modern-love-to-fall-in-love-with-anyone-do-this.html

Clatichi, V. G. (2020, July 11). How long does it actually take to form a new habit? Backed by science! Www.linkedin.com. https://www.linkedin.com/pulse/how-long-does-actually-take-form-new-habit-backed-science-clatici

Duhigg, C. (2011). How habits work - Charles Duhigg. Charles Duhigg. https://charlesduhigg.com/how-habits-work/

Duhigg, C. (2013). The power of habit : Why we do what we do and how to change. Random House.

Glover Tawwab, N. (2021). Set boundaries, find peace : A guide to reclaiming yourself. Penguin Publishing Group.

Goodreads. (n.d.-a). A quote by Bob Marley. Www.goodreads.com. Retrieved April 8, 2022, from https://www.goodreads.com/quotes/93997-love-the-life-you-live-live-the-life-you-love

Goodreads. (n.d.-b). A quote by Lucille Ball. Www.goodreads.com. Retrieved April 7, 2022, from https://www.goodreads.com/quotes/16342-love-yourself-first-and-everything-else-falls-into-line-your

Goodreads. (n.d.-c). A quote by Rumi. Www.goodreads.com. Retrieved April 7, 2022, from https://www.goodreads.com/quotes/9726-your-task-is-not-to-seek-for-love-but-merely

Goodreads. (n.d.-d). A quote by Socrates. Www.goodreads.com. Retrieved March 16, 2022, from https://www.goodreads.com/quotes/398845-my-friend-care-for-your-psyche-know-thyself-for-once-we-know

Goodreads. (n.d.-e). A quote by Victor Hugo. Www.goodreads.com. Retrieved April 8, 2022, from https://www.goodreads.com/quotes/19349-the-greatest-happiness-of-life-is-the-conviction-that-we

Goodreads. (n.d.-f). A quote from the perks of being a wallflower. Www.goodreads.com. https://www.goodreads.com/quotes/2534-we-accept-the-love-we-think-we-deserve

Gottman, J. M., & Silver, N. (2018). The seven principles for making marriage work. Seven Dials An Imprint Of Orion Publishing Group Ltd.

Harvard Health Publishing. (2020, July 7). Exercising to relax - Harvard health. Harvard Health; Harvard Health. https://www.health.harvard.edu/staying-healthy/exercising-to-relax

Krawczyk, D. C. (2018). Social Cognition. Reasoning, 10(1016), 283–311. https://doi.org/10.1016/b978-0-12-809285-9.00012-0

Krznaric, R. (2015). Empathy : Why it matters, and how to get it. Perigee.

Lewis, T., Amini, F., & Lannon, R. (2001). A general theory of love. Vintage Books.

Love Expands. (2019, August 20). You'll be amazed at what you attract when you start believing in what you deserve. Love Expands. https://loveexpands.com/youll-be-amazed-at-what-you-attract-when-you-start-believing-in-what-you-deserve/

McLachlan, S. (2021, December 22). The science of habit: How to rewire your brain. Healthline. https://www.healthline.com/health/the-science-of-habit#4

Mclaren, K. (2013). The art of empathy : A complete guide to life's most essential skill. Sounds True, Inc.

Morgan, C. T., King, R. A., & Weisz, J. R. (2010). Introduction to psychology. Tata Mcgraw-Hill Publishing Co. Ltd.

Quote Catalog. (n.d.). Roy Croft quote - I love you not because of who you are, b... | Quote Catalog. Quotecatalog.com. Retrieved April 7, 2022, from https://quotecatalog.com/quote/roy-croft-i-love-you-not-zpW50g1

Quote Fancy. (n.d.). Nicky James Quote: "Don't confuse your path with your destination. Just because it's stormy now doesn't mean that you aren't headed for suns..." Quotefancy.com. Retrieved April 7, 2022, from https://quotefancy.com/quote/2880792/Nicky-James-Don-t-confuse-your-path-with-your-destination-Just-because-it-s-stormy-now

Raypole, C. (2021, February 5). Habit loop: What it is and how to break it. Healthline. https://www.healthline.com/health/mental-health/habit-loop#components

Reader's Digest Editors. (2021, December 23). The 36 questions that can lead to love. Reader's Digest. https://www.rd.com/list/arthur-aron-36-questions/

Ryan, R. M., & Deci, E. L. (2017). Self-determination theory : Basic psychological needs in motivation, development, and wellness. Guilford Press.

Segar, M. (2015). No sweat : How the simple science of motivation can bring you a lifetime of fitness. Amacom--American Management Association.

Teixeira, P. J., Silva, M. N., Mata, J., Palmeira, A. L., & Markland, D. (2012). Motivation, self-determination, and long-term weight control. International Journal of Behavioral Nutrition and Physical Activity, 9(1), 22. https://doi.org/10.1186/1479-5868-9-22

The Extension. (n.d.). Some of our favorite recovery quotes – the extension. Theextension.org. Retrieved April 8, 2022, from https://theextension.org/some-of-our-favorite-recovery-quotes/#:~:text=At%20the%20end%20of%20life

Tiny Buddha. (n.d.). Love is not what you say. Love is what you do. Tiny Buddha. Retrieved April 7, 2022, from https://tinybuddha.com/wisdom-quotes/love-not-say-love/

US Department of Health and Human Services. (2016, November). The neurobiology of substance use, misuse, and addiction. Nih.gov; US Department of Health and Human Services. https://www.ncbi.nlm.nih.gov/books/NBK424849/

Wood, W. (2019). Good habits, bad habits : The science of making positive changes that stick. Macmillan An Imprint Of Pan Macmillan.

CDC. (2020, September 8). *Adverse Childhood Experiences (ACEs)*. www.cdc.gov. https://www.cdc.gov/violenceprevention/aces/index.html

Davis, S. (2020, July 20). *Healing Trauma Through Inner Child Work*. C-PTSD Foundation. https://cptsdfoundation.org/2020/07/20/healing-trauma-through-inner-child-work/

Davis, S. (2021, May 24). *Changing the Future by Acknowledging the Past*. C-PTSD Foundation. https://cptsdfoundation.org/2021/05/24/changing-the-future-by-acknowledging-the-past/

Gilles, G. (2018, January 26). *Complex PTSD: Symptoms, tests, treatment, and finding support*. Healthline.

https://www.healthline.com/health/cptsd#:~:text=Similarly%2C%20people%20with%20PTSD%20have

Harvard Health Publishing. (2020, July 6). *Understanding the Stress Response*. Harvard Health; Harvard Health. https://www.health.harvard.edu/staying-healthy/understanding-the-stress-response

LaSov, A. (2020, February 4). *How to Live With Complex PTSD*. Advekit. https://www.advekit.com/blogs/how-to-live-with-complex-ptsd

NHS. (2021, February 17). *Complex PTSD—Post-traumatic Stress Disorder*. Nhs.uk. https://www.nhs.uk/mental-health/conditions/post-traumatic-stress-disorder-ptsd/complex/

Elliot, A. J. (2015). Color and Psychological Functioning: A Review of Theoretical and Empirical Work. *Frontiers in Psychology, 6*(368). https://doi.org/10.3389/fpsyg.2015.00368

Gilles, G. (2018, January 26). *Understanding Complex Post-Traumatic Stress Disorder*. Healthline; Healthline Media. https://www.healthline.com/health/cptsd

Goleman, D. (1995). *Emotional Intelligence: Why It Can Matter More Than IQ*. Bloomsbury.

Pattemore, C. (2021, June 3). *10 Ways to Build and Preserve Better Boundaries*. Psych Central. https://psychcentral.com/lib/10-way-to-build-and-preserve-better-boundaries

QuoteFancy. (n.d.-a). *John Callahan quote: "Sex is like air; it's not important unless you aren't getting any."* Quotefancy.com. Retrieved March 9, 2022, from https://quotefancy.com/quote/37107/John-Callahan-Sex-is-like-air-it-s-not-important-unless-you-aren-t-getting-any

QuoteFancy. (n.d.-b). *John Green quote: "The darkest nights produce the brightest stars."* Quotefancy.com. Retrieved

March 9, 2022, from https://quotefancy.com/quote/843318/John-Green-The-darkest-nights-produce-the-brightest-stars#:~:text=John%20Green%20Quote%3A%20%E2%80%9CThe%20darkest

Raypole, C. (2020, September 23). *Toxic Shame: What It Is and How to Cope*. Healthline. https://www.healthline.com/health/mental-health/toxic-shame#working-through-it

Rowling, J. K. (2014). *Harry Potter and the Prisoner of Azkaban*. Bloomsbury.

Yeo, A. (2016, February 24). *The Story of Two Wolves*. Urban Balance. https://www.urbanbalance.com/the-story-of-two-wolves/

www.ingramcontent.com/pod-product-compliance
Lightning Source LLC
Chambersburg PA
CBHW060317030426
42336CB00011B/1092
9781778275425